INTRODUCTION

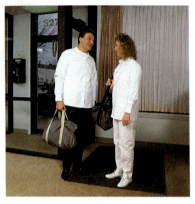

Welcome to the cosmetology profession.

Here you are at the threshold of opportunity. You have a chance for glamour, excitement, and other untold rewards. Welcome to the world of cosmetology! Apply yourself and there are no limits to the possibilities. Your license to practice cosmetology is an unlimited passport to the world.

Whether you like working with hair, skin, or nails, your certification provides you with the opportunity to select a career path to suit you. To get the most out of your passport, make the most of your education. Every lesson has something to teach you, something that may start you on your way. Your license unlocks countless doors, but it is what *you learn* that can really launch your career.

THE WORLD OF COSMETOLOGY

As you begin your journey, you may not know whether you prefer working with hair, skin, or nails. Even if you do have something in mind, leave yourself open to other possibilities. Let your learning guide you. Enter each classroom with an open mind and a wholehearted desire to learn as much as you can.

Some of the most well-known people in the beauty world began just as you are beginning. A broad beauty education gave them the chance to enthusiastically explore different avenues of cosmetology until they found the path that suited them. Why not give yourself that chance as well? You have so many possibilities. Here are just some of the many vocations that you may be tempted to try upon graduation. No matter what area interests you, take the time to read the following sections. Each one has helpful information suggested by some of the most accomplished professionals in the beauty world today.

MAKEUP ARTIST

Are you artistically inclined? Do you like blending, shading, creating? A makeup artist "paints faces," explains one top artist in the field. "He or she brings out beauty without making it look like a disguise." Makeup artists most frequently apply cosmetics to enhance a client's appearance, but they can create *any* image a particular job calls for.

As a makeup artist, you can establish yourself in a salon with a private clientele, become makeup director for a prestigious department store, represent a line of cosmetics, work in television and movie production, find a position with a fashion magazine, or work behind the scenes in theater production. You can operate as an independent freelancer, which allows you to create your own schedule, or you can find full-time employment with one company.

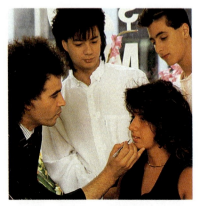

Makeup artist.

Advice from the Experts

"Makeup artistry is so much more than just fashion and taste. It's a lot of training," advises a top talent in the field. "If you don't learn as much as you can, eventually it corners you." Pay strict attention in *all* your classes. Concentrate on chemistry and anatomy.

After beauty school, consider continuing your education in the fine arts, with an emphasis on drawing and painting courses. Theater experience will also prove helpful, especially a study of stage lighting.

Work in a salon for at least six months after school. Consider volunteering your services to community theaters, fashion shows, and department stores in your area. Volunteer work will afford you experience and help you build a resume as well as contacts, that is, people you meet who may be important to your career. Start to develop a portfolio that you can present to potential employers. In this portfolio, compile before and after photographs of makeovers you have performed, along with any awards or certificates you may have earned.

SKIN CARE SPECIALIST/ESTHETICIAN

Are you drawn by the allure of a radiant complexion and the secrets of different creams and lotions? An *esthetician* offers treatments to perfect the look and health of skin.

As an esthetician you can work in a salon, teach, travel throughout the world giving demonstrations at beauty shows, or become a consultant to a cosmetic company. You can work exclusively for one company or you can be a freelancer.

Advice from the Experts

Consider attending a beauty school that specializes in or emphasizes facial treatments. "Devote yourself to your training," advises an esthetician who lectures worldwide. "It's such a short training period and once you start work, it's difficult to get away to take classes."

Read as much as you can about skin care. "Since I was always reading, I could sound authoritative when I spoke to clients," continues the skin care expert. Attend seminars where you can meet and learn from the specialists in your area of interest. Subscribe to professional publications that list events and classes you can participate in to supplement your education. Study the different skin care products on the market so that you understand what they are supposed to do and how you can use them.

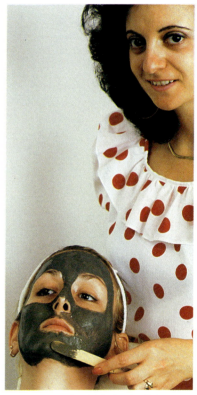

Skin care specialist/esthetician.

COSMETIC CHEMIST

Are you curious and creative? Do you like experimenting? Cosmetic chemists supply the beauty world's expanding needs by creating new products through research and experimentation.

"Every business has its tools," explains one cosmetic chemist. "I help make the tools that cosmetologists use." He continues, "I get a profile from the marketing company that shows what type of product they want to market. Then I go through my mental and physical library to bring together that product."

As a cosmetic chemist you can work for a cosmetic manufacturer or become a consultant to several companies.

Advice from the Experts

Learn everything you can in cosmetology school. "I draw from everything I've studied," confirms one highly paid cosmetic chemist. Pay close attention to your marketing courses. An understanding of the commercial marketplace will help to direct your scientific exploration. It is also important to acquire a chemistry education in addition to what you learn in beauty school. You should consider continuing your education in a college.

After completing your schooling, apply for an internship with a cosmetic company working on a panel that studies new products. If you can't get into a company this way, apply for a position in the manufacturer's marketing department.

PUBLISHING

Do you like to write? You can use your cosmetology license to enter the publishing world. With a beauty background, you can write articles, books, brochures, columns, educational manuals—even produce videos. "You get to wear the latest, trendiest hairstyles, clothes, and accessories *and* you get to do what you love," says one cosmetologist turned beauty writer.

As a writer with a cosmetology license, you can work for a publishing company, freelance, travel and review major beauty shows, or develop a lifestyle that combines it all.

Advice from the Experts

Master the technical basics of cosmetology. "You need to really understand *why* a certain procedure works better in order to write about it," explains one cosmetology editor with a major publishing firm. "It's a way to open doors. Then, you can go on to let your creativity out."

Fine-tune your writing skills by taking writing courses and reading as much as possible to see how things are written.

Keep current with what's happening in your industry by attending seminars. "You can use this knowledge to determine what to write, because you'll know what's needed," advises the publishing expert. "Be up on the latest information because you can bet your audience will be."

Practice networking; create contacts by being open and friendly with other people. These contacts might have a hot tip for you or remember your name when a position opens.

HAIRCOLORIST

Do you have an exacting eye for pigment? Do flattering shades jump out at you? A haircolorist picks out the best color and process to enhance a client's hair. The colorist mixes the dye, applies it, and evaluates the resulting shade.

"Haircoloring is such a creative part of the industry," says one noted haircolorist. "There's so many different ways to arrive at a color. It's not like haircutting where there's only one way."

As a haircolorist you can establish a specialized color department within a salon, become a color trainer (teaching at salons), work for a haircolor manufacturer, or become a **platform artist**, demonstrating your technique at national and international shows.

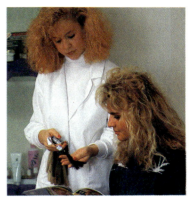

Haircolorist.

Advice from the Experts

Persevere and pay attention in beauty school. Take advantage of opportunities to work with your teachers. For example, ask if you can assist with a coloring. Observe other teachers or students doing color as often as you can. Attend classes and shows in your area. Most important, keep practicing. "Don't be afraid to make mistakes," advises one haircolorist. "You're going to make mistakes. It's the first ten thousand that are the toughest. Just keep going."

SALON OWNER

Do you have great ideas for how things *should* be done? Do you like varied responsibilities and challenges? Running your own salon allows you to set a standard for the quality of service you bring to the marketplace. You can choose the products and services to provide, and establish the level of skill you demand from your staff. You can exercise creativity, versatility, and independence in this position if you don't mind making decisions and putting in long hours.

Advice from the Experts

In beauty school you must learn everything you possibly can, paying particular attention to sales courses. When you graduate, take a job as a cosmetologist. "Never come right out and own a salon," says one salon owner of eighteen years. "A school environment is totally different from a salon. You absolutely need to work for a while first."

Owning a salon means assuming responsibility for paying bills, payrolls, and taxes as much as it means doing nails and giving haircuts and perms. You must develop business skills beyond what you learn in beauty school. Attend college business classes or seminars. You might even want to attend business school. You should also contact your local small business bureau and obtain literature about businesses in your area. Talk to local salon owners and learn what you can from their experience.

In addition to business expertise, you need people skills to run a salon. You will be in the public's eye and you will be managing a staff of employees. Take some courses that build upon your social skills and suggest successful techniques for resolving conflicts.

RETAIL SPECIALIST

Do you have a flair for selling? Do you communicate well and enjoy working with people? With a cosmetology license, you can become a retail specialist working with salons and manufacturers to promote their products' sales. "Retailing is nothing more than good communication," explains one retail specialist who lectures nationwide. "All you need to do is understand people enough to sell your product, your service, and yourself."

As a retail specialist, you can work in a salon, spa, or department store as a product manager handling the merchandising of inventory. Retail specialists also work as trainers, honing the sales techniques of a particular cosmetic company, or traveling throughout the country presenting general sales seminars. "Being a retail specialist is a great security," advises a self-made retail specialist. "Even as a stylist, every salon will want to hire you. You know a lot about sales, and salons today have to focus on sales."

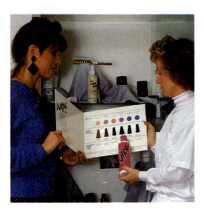
Retail specialist.

Advice from the Experts

Get the best technological understanding you can at beauty school. To really sell a product, you need to know how to work with it and why it stands out as a product you recommend.

Work for a salon after beauty school. Time "in the trenches" gives you the experience you will need to market yourself to companies as an authority whom they can trust. Read about selling strategies. Spend time observing people. "If you don't understand people, you don't understand the business," advises one retail specialist, who recommends drawing from past work experience and practicing people skills daily.

COMPETITION CHAMPION

Are you a perfectionist? Do you get excited working toward a goal and winning? Competition champions compete for prizes and prestige in various cosmetology world championships. Here, "the best" display their individual talents and techniques. You must have dedication, good work habits, and utmost skill to enter this honored realm that holds so many rewards.

"The commitment reflects on your everyday lifestyle," explains one champion who has competed for years. "As you train to be a winner, you bring back that attitude to the salon. You have no limit to what you can do."

Competition champions often establish their own salons. Their reputation as distinguished artists attracts a following and adds to the prosperity of their business endeavors. Champions can also work as trainers, coaching the next generation of competitors.

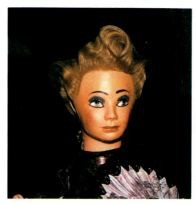

Competition winner.

Advice from the Experts

In beauty school, make sure you cultivate your styling skills as perfectly as possible. Pay close attention to details. Make sure everything is balanced and immaculate. "Your combing should be spotless," advises one champion who now trains competitors. "Walk around the client and look at your work from different angles."

To enter competitions, you may need to hire a world champion trainer, spend time creating and perfecting your skills, and search for the right model. But for those dedicated to the path, the reward can be exhilaration and prestige.

EDUCATIONAL SPECIALIST

Do you like to teach? Do you enjoy seeing people grasp new information? The beauty industry abounds in teaching opportunities. For example, an educational consultant who works for a product manufacturer might conduct seminars for a salon staff, demonstrating how to use various products. Other consultants work for manufacturers of ingredients that are sold to cosmetic companies. They give presentations to the marketing departments of cosmetic companies to demonstrate how an ingredient can improve or enhance a product.

Other educational specialists write curriculums and training manuals that teach consultants to teach. As an educational specialist, you might work for a major manufacturer or travel around the country training industry professionals to teach.

Advice from the Experts

Concentrate on all your courses in beauty school. "All skills become cumulative," explains one educational specialist on board with a major manufacturer. "You may not like to do manicures, but it's always another skill you can pose to an employer to get your foot in the door of a job you want." Since marketing goes hand in hand with the educational specialist's objectives, consider adding some business courses to your training.

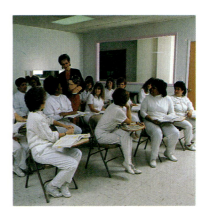

Educator.

Yet another way to begin your career is by working in a major department store training sales clerks to demonstrate and sell cosmetics. Then, prepare your resume and mail it to every manufacturer you can think of, outlining your skills, experience, and the type of position you are seeking.

The list of career opportunities is endless. The beauty industry continues to grow in order to accommodate the vivid imaginations and abilities of the artists. Welcome to this wonderful world of possibilities where, if you can imagine your ideal career, with a little perseverance, you can probably spend your life doing it!

YOUR PROFESSIONAL IMAGE

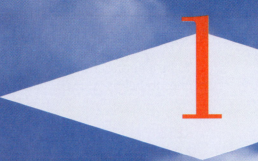

LEARNING OBJECTIVES

AFTER COMPLETING THIS CHAPTER, YOU SHOULD BE ABLE TO:

1. Demonstrate guidelines to maintain a healthy body and mind.
2. List the qualities of effective physical presentation.
3. Define personality.
4. List the qualities of effective communication.
5. Demonstrate good human relations and a professional attitude.
6. Define professional ethics.

INTRODUCTION

Good health is a basic element for living. Without it, one cannot work efficiently or enjoy the pleasures of life. As a cosmetologist, you should be a living example of good health so that you increase your value to yourself, to your employer, and to the community.

YOUR PERSONAL AND PROFESSIONAL HEALTH

To be a successful cosmetologist, you should follow a set of guidelines to help you maintain a healthy body and mind.

REST

Adequate sleep is essential for good health. Without it you cannot function efficiently. The body should be allowed to recover from the fatigue of the day's activities and should be replenished with a good night's sleep. The amount of sleep needed to feel refreshed varies from person to person. Some people function well with 6 hours of sleep; others need 8 hours.

EXERCISE

Exercise ensures the proper functioning of organs such as the heart and lungs, strengthens muscles and bones, and improves circulation. An adequate fitness program includes exercises to accomplish aerobic strength, flexibility, and endurance.

RELAXATION

Relaxation is important as a change of pace from your day-to-day routine. Going to a movie or a museum, reading a book, watching television, or dancing are ways for you to "get away from it all." When you return to work, you will feel refreshed and eager to attend to your duties.

NUTRITION

What you eat affects your health, appearance, personality, and performance on the job. The nutrients in food supply the body with energy and ensure proper body functions. A balanced diet should include a variety of foods so that you obtain important vitamins and minerals. Drink plenty of water daily. Try to avoid sugar, salt, caffeine, and fatty or highly refined and processed foods and "fast" foods.

PERSONAL HYGIENE

Personal hygiene is the daily maintenance of cleanliness and healthfulness. The basics include daily bathing or showering, using deodorant, brushing your teeth and using mouthwash to freshen your breath during the day, and having clean and well-groomed hair and nails.

PERSONAL GROOMING

Personal grooming is an extension of personal hygiene. A well-groomed cosmetologist is one of the best advertisements for a salon. If you present a poised and attractive image, your client will have confidence in you as a professional. Many salon owners and managers consider appearance, personality, and poise to be as important as technical knowledge and manual skills. To begin, wear fresh undergarments daily and a freshly laundered, well-tailored uniform. Some salons do not require standard uniforms, but they may have a specific dress code. For example, some salons require that all their personnel wear the same color clothing. Select your outfits so that you reflect the image of the salon. Avoid obtrusive or excessive jewelry. A wristwatch will help you keep to your schedule.

The Female Cosmetologist

The female cosmetologist should wear stylish shoes that fit and are still comfortable at the end of a long day. Your makeup should be flattering and suited to the environment of your salon. (Fig. 1.1)

The Male Cosmetologist

In addition to the general guidelines discussed, the male cosmetologist should keep facial hair neatly trimmed and groomed. (Fig. 1.2)

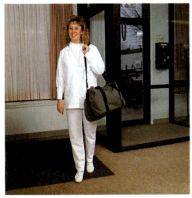

1.1—A well-groomed female cosmetologist.

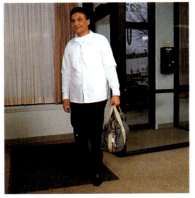

1.2—A well-groomed male cosmetologist.

CARE OF THE FEET

As a cosmetologist you will spend a great deal of time on your feet. Proper foot care will help you maintain a good posture and a cheerful attitude. Sore feet or poor-fitting shoes can cause great discomfort. (Fig. 1.3)

Shoes

Try to wear shoes with low, broad heels and with cushioned insoles. They give you support and balance, which help to maintain good posture and offset fatigue that can result from hours of standing. It also helps if you can stand on a carpeted or cushioned surface.

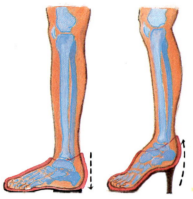

1.3—For comfort and to help maintain good posture, wear well-fitted, low-heeled shoes.

Daily Foot Care

After bathing, apply cream or oil and massage each foot for 5 minutes. Remove the cream or oil and apply an antiseptic foot lotion. Regular pedicures that include cleansing, removal of calloused skin, massage, and toenail trims will keep your feet at their best. When your feet ache, podiatrists recommend that you soak your feet alternately in warm and cool water. See a podiatrist if corns, bunions, ingrown toenails, or other foot disorders exist.

Professional Prep

DRESSING FOR SUCCESS

Whether or not a salon has a dress code or grooming policy, a stylist should always look his or her best—and should fit in with the clientele. (If your clients are conservative, save your trendiest, most outrageous outfits and hairstyles for your days off.) If uniforms are required by your salon, make sure yours is crisp and clean at all times.

A male stylist who wears a shirt and tie not only looks more professional, but can demand more money. Female stylists should wear clean, run-free hose, and be sure their slips are not showing. Jewelry should be simple and attractive.

All female stylists should have their hair done at least once a week, and their hair should reflect the best workmanship of the salon. Hair coloring should be encouraged, and if the salon specializes in wigs or other artificial hair, the stylists should wear them at work. Male employees should have haircuts twice a month, in attractive and moderate styles. They should shave every day, and if they wear a beard it should be trimmed regularly.

Makeup should be worn by all female stylists, but in moderation. Too much makeup is inappropriate in a work setting.

Shoes must be clean and neat at all times. Rundown heels are very hard on the feet when standing all day. No one should be allowed to work with dirty shoes.

—*From* Salon Management for Cosmetology Students *by Edward Tezak*

HEALTHY LIFESTYLE

You should practice stress management through relaxation, rest, and exercise and avoid substances that can negatively affect your good health, such as cigarettes, alcohol, and drugs. ✔

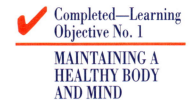

✓ Completed—Learning Objective No. 1

MAINTAINING A HEALTHY BODY AND MIND

PHYSICAL PRESENTATION

Your posture, walk, and movements all make up your physical presentation. People form opinions about you by the way you present yourself. Do you stand straight or slouch; do you walk confidently or do you drag your feet? Your physical presentation is part of your professional image.

GOOD POSTURE

Good posture not only improves your personal appearance by presenting your figure to advantage and creating an image of confidence, it also prevents fatigue and many other physical problems. (Figs. 1.4, 1.5) Because you will be spending most of your time on your feet when working as a professional cosmetologist, good posture should be developed as early as possible through regular exercise and self-discipline.

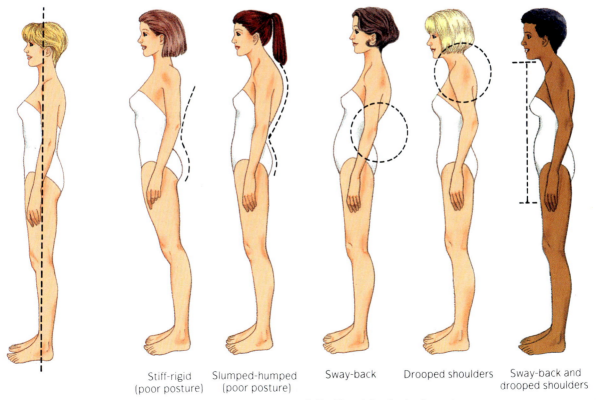

Stiff-rigid (poor posture)   Slumped-humped (poor posture)   Sway-back   Drooped shoulders   Sway-back and drooped shoulders

1.4—Good posture.   1.5—Five defective body postures.

PHYSICAL PRESENTATION ON THE JOB

To prevent muscle aches, back strain, discomfort, fatigue, and other problems and to maintain an attractive image, it is very important to practice good physical presentation while performing work activities. (Figs. 1.6, 1.7)

Checkpoints of Good Posture

- Crown of head reaching upward while chin is kept level with the floor.
- Neck is elongated and balanced directly above the shoulders.
- Chest up; body is lifted from the breastbone.
- Shoulders are level, held back and down, yet relaxed.
- Spine is straight, not curved laterally or swayed from front to back.
- Abdomen is flat.
- Hips are level (horizontally) and protrude neither forward nor back.
- Knees are slightly flexed and positioned directly over the feet with the ankles firm.

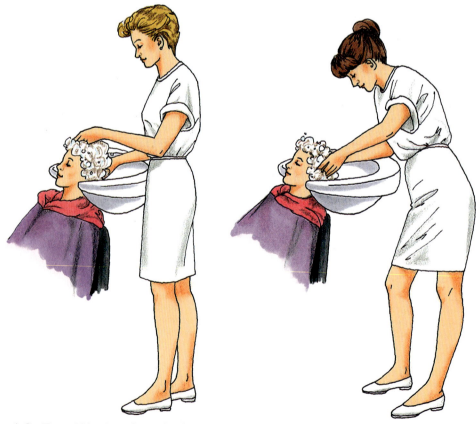

1.6—To avoid back strain, maintain good posture when giving a shampoo.

1.7—Poor posture.

Basic Stance for Women

- Place most of your weight on your right foot and point your toes straight ahead in a straight line.
- Place your left heel close to the heel or instep of your right foot and point the toes slightly outward.
- Bend your left knee slightly inward. (Fig. 1.8)

Basic Stance for Men

- Place your feet apart, but not wider than your shoulder width.
- Distribute your weight evenly over both feet.
- Your knees should be neither rigid nor bent.
- Your toes should point straight ahead or one or both feet should point slightly outward.
- For a more relaxed stance, bend one knee slightly while shifting some of your weight to the opposite foot. (Fig. 1.9)

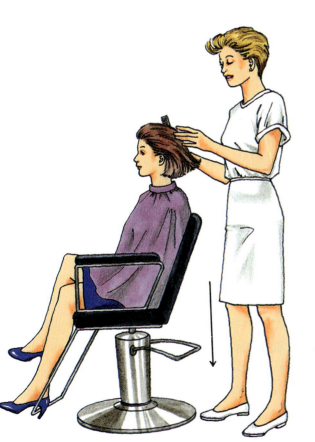
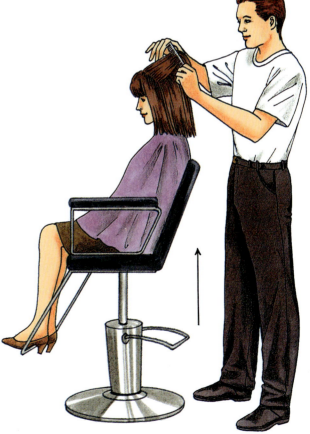

1.8—Basic stance for the female cosmetologist, and the correct chair position for working on a client comfortably.

1.9—Basic stance for the male cosmetologist, and the correct chair position for working on a client comfortably.

CORRECT SITTING TECHNIQUE

To sit attractively, use your thigh muscles and support from your hands and arms to lower your body smoothly into a chair. Do not fall or flop into a chair. When lowering your body, keep your back straight. Do not bend at the waist or reach with the buttocks. When seated, slide to the back of the chair by placing both hands on the front edge of the chair at the sides of your hips. Raise your body slightly and slide back. Do not wiggle or inch back.

When giving a manicure, assume a correct sitting position. Sit with the lower back against the chair, leaning slightly forward. If a stool is used, sit on the entire stool. Keep your chest up and rest your body weight on the full length of your thighs. (Figs. 1.10, 1.11)

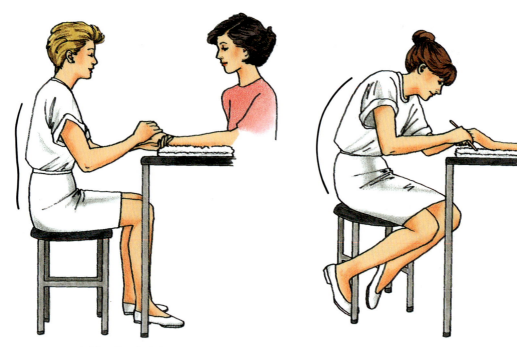

1.10—Good sitting posture.   1.11—Poor sitting posture.

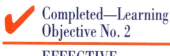

Completed—Learning Objective No. 2

EFFECTIVE PHYSICAL PRESENTATION

Tips for a Proper Sitting Position
1. Keep your feet close together.
2. Keep your knees close together.
3. Place your feet out slightly farther than your knees.
4. Do not push your feet under the chair.
5. Keep the entire sole of your foot on the floor. ✔

PERSONALITY

Your personality plays an important part in your personal and professional life. Personality can be defined as the outward reflection of your inner feelings, thoughts, attitudes, and values. Your personality is expressed through your voice, speech, and choice of words, as well as through your facial expressions, gestures, actions, posture, clothing, grooming, and environment. It is the total effect you have on other people.

DESIRABLE QUALITIES FOR EFFECTIVE CLIENT RELATIONS

Emotional Control

Learn to control your emotions. Discourage and do not reveal negative emotions such as anger, envy, and dislike. An even-tempered person is always treated with respect.

Positive Approach

Be pleasant and gracious. A smile of greeting and a word of welcome should be ready for each client and co-worker. A good sense of humor is also an important part of maintaining a positive attitude. A sense of humor enriches your life and cushions the disappointments. When you are able to laugh at yourself, you will have gained the ability to accept and deal positively with difficult situations.

Good Manners

Good manners reflect your thoughtfulness of others. Saying "thank you" and "please," treating other people with respect, exercising care of other people's property, being tolerant and understanding of other people's shortcomings and efforts, and being considerate of those with whom you work all express good manners. Courtesy is one of the keys to a successful career.

Bad Manners

Gum chewing and nervous habits such as tapping your foot or playing with your hair and personal items detract from your effectiveness. Yawning, coughing, and sneezing should be concealed when in the presence of others. Control body language that reveals negative communication, for example, sarcastic or disapproving facial grimaces. Pleasant facial expressions and attractive gestures and actions should be your goal. ✔

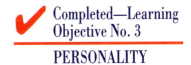

Completed—Learning Objective No. 3

PERSONALITY

EFFECTIVE COMMUNICATION

Communication includes your listening skills, voice, speech, manner of speaking, and conversational skills. Your ability to communicate will have a great influence on your effectiveness as a cosmetologist. A cosmetologist needs good communication skills for the following reasons:

- To make contacts
- To meet and greet clients
- To understand a client's needs, likes, dislikes, and desires (Fig. 1.12)
- To be self-promoting
- To sell services and products (Fig. 1.13)
- To build business
- To talk on the telephone
- To carry on a pleasant conversation
- To interact with the salon staff

✓ Completed—Learning Objective No. 4
EFFECTIVE COMMUNICATION

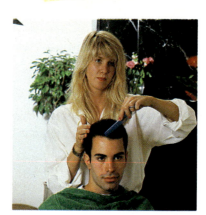

1.12—Cosmetologist communicating with client.

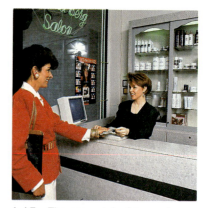

1.13—The cosmetologist as salesperson.

HUMAN RELATIONS AND YOUR PROFESSIONAL ATTITUDE

Human relations is the psychology of getting along well with others. Your professional attitude is expressed by your own self-esteem, confidence in your profession, and by the respect you show others.

Good habits and practices acquired during your school training lay the foundation for a successful career in cosmetology. The following are guidelines for good human relations that will help you to gain confidence and deal successfully with others.

1. Always greet a client by name, with a pleasant tone of voice. Address a client by his or her last name (Mrs. Smith, Mr. Jones, Miss Allen) unless the client prefers first names and it is customary to use first names in your salon.
2. Be alert to the client's mood. Some clients prefer quiet and relaxation, others like to talk. Be a good listener and confine your conversation to the client's needs. Never gossip or tell off-color stories. (Fig. 1.14)
3. Topics of conversation should be carefully chosen. Friendly relations are achieved through pleasant conversations. Let your client be the guide in the topic of conversation. In a business setting it is best to avoid discussing controversial topics such as religion and politics, topics that relate to your personal life such as personal problems, or subjects relating to other people such as another client's behavior, poor workmanship of fellow workers or competitors, or information given to you in confidence.
4. Make a good impression by looking the part of the successful cosmetologist, and by speaking and acting in a professional manner at all times.
5. Cultivate self-confidence, and project a pleasing personality.
6. Show interest in the client's personal preferences. Give your undivided attention. Maintain eye contact and concentrate totally on your client.
7. Use tact and diplomacy when dealing with problems you may encounter.
8. Be capable and efficient in your work.
9. Be punctual. Arrive at work on time and keep appointments on schedule. Plan each day's schedule so that you manage your time effectively.
10. Develop your business and sales abilities. Use tact when suggesting additional services or products to clients.
11. Avoid saying anything that sounds as if you are criticizing, condemning, or putting down a client's opinions.
12. Keep informed of new products and services so you can answer clients' questions intelligently.
13. Continue to add to your knowledge and skills.
14. Be ethical in all your dealings with clients and others with whom you come in contact.
15. Always let the client see that you practice the highest standards of sanitation.
16. Avoid criticizing your competitors.
17. Deal with all disputes and differences in private. Take care of all problems promptly.

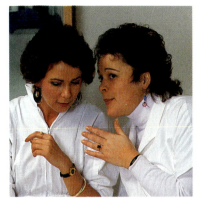

1.14—Nobody likes a person who gossips.

Professional Prep

HONING YOUR PEOPLE SKILLS

Every business that provides services to people must deal with clients who are rude, pushy, upset, angry, hostile, selfish, deceitful, critical, and manipulative. These people all fall into a category labeled "difficult." How can you deal effectively with difficult people? Here are some tips:

Accept people as they are. Remember, you can't change another person's behavior. What you can change is the way you react to that person. Stop allowing other people's behavior to affect or influence you.

Ask questions to clarify and summarize. Only after the upset or angry person has had a chance to get the problem off his or her chest, calmly ask open-ended questions.

Refrain from becoming emotional. No matter what, you can't allow yourself to be drawn into the emotional part of the problem. You must remain cool and calm, pleasant and professional. You must think objectively, not emotionally.

Work on feeling good about yourself. People with low self-esteem are more vulnerable to difficult people and their tactics. Concentrate on being positive and upbeat. Think positive thoughts and make positive statements.

—From *Communication Skills for Cosmetologists* by Kathleen Ann Bergant

TO BE SUCCESSFUL...

1. Be punctual. Get to work on time and keep all appointments. Being punctual gains the admiration and confidence of your clients, your manager, and your co-workers.
2. Be courteous. Courtesy plays an important part in bringing clients to the salon and in keeping them as regular customers.
3. Set a good example for your profession. Your own neat, attractive, and fashionable appearance expresses your pride in yourself and your profession. Clients have confidence in the cosmetologist who looks the part.
4. Be efficient and skillful. Practice your skills so that you can give services efficiently and gently. Clients appreciate the cosmetologist who cares about their comfort and is skillful when giving services.
5. Practice effective communications. Speaking well of others and being able to give sincere compliments will be an asset in your career as a professional cosmetologist. Being a good listener and being efficient and courteous when speaking on the telephone or with clients during the service will help you build a successful business.

To be successful, you should extend courtesy to all with whom you come in contact. This includes state board members and inspectors, who are contributing to the higher standards of cosmetology.

To be successful, you must know the laws, rules, and regulations that govern cosmetology, and you must comply with them. By complying, you are contributing to the health, welfare, and safety of your community. ✔

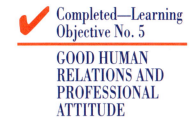

Completed—Learning Objective No. 5

GOOD HUMAN RELATIONS AND PROFESSIONAL ATTITUDE

PROFESSIONAL ETHICS

Ethics is defined as the study of standards of conduct and moral judgment. Codes of ethics for various professions are established by boards or commissions. In cosmetology, each state has a board or commission that sets standards that all cosmetologists who work in that state must follow. However, ethics goes beyond a set of rules and regulations. In the field of cosmetology, ethics is also a code of behavior by which you conduct yourself. Much of what was discussed in the previous section is directly related to an informal code of ethical standards.

Ethics deal with proper conduct and business dealings with employers, clients and co-workers, and others with whom you come in contact. Ethical conduct helps to build the client's confidence in you. Having your clients speak well of you to others is the best form of advertising and helps you build a successful business. The following are rules of ethics you should practice:

1. Give courteous and friendly service to all clients. Treat everyone honestly and fairly; do not show favoritism.
2. Be courteous and show respect for the feelings, beliefs, and rights of others.
3. Keep your word. Be responsible and fulfill your obligations.
4. Build your reputation by setting an example of good conduct and behavior.
5. Be loyal to your employer, managers, and associates.
6. Obey all provisions of the state cosmetology laws.
7. Practice the highest standards of sanitation to protect your health and the health of your co-workers and clients.
8. Believe in the cosmetology profession. Practice it faithfully and sincerely.
9. Do not try to sell your clients a product or service they do not need or want.
10. As a student:
    - Be loyal to, and cooperate with, school personnel and fellow students.
    - Comply with school and clinic rules and regulations.

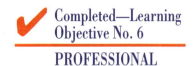

Completed—Learning Objective No. 6

PROFESSIONAL ETHICS

Questionable practices, extravagant claims, and unfulfilled promises violate the rules of ethical conduct and cast an unfavorable light on cosmetology. Unethical practices affect the student, the cosmetologist, the school or salon, and the entire industry. ✔

REVIEW QUESTIONS

YOUR PROFESSIONAL IMAGE

1. List the guidelines you should follow to maintain a healthy body and mind. *page 10-13*
2. Define physical presentation. *page 13*
3. Define personality. *page 17*
4. What does communication consist of? *page 18*
5. Define good human relations. *page 18*
6. How is your professional attitude expressed? *page 18*
7. What is professional ethics? *page 21*

BACTERIOLOGY

2

LEARNING OBJECTIVES

AFTER COMPLETING THIS CHAPTER, YOU SHOULD BE ABLE TO:

1. List the various types and classifications of bacteria.
2. Describe how bacteria grow and reproduce.
3. Describe the relationship of bacteria to the spread of disease.
4. Define AIDS and provide brief overview of AIDS.

INTRODUCTION

Bacteriology (bak-teer-ee-**OL**-o-jee), *sterilization* (ster-il-ih-**ZAY**-shun), and *sanitation* (san-ih-**TAY**-shun) are subjects of practical importance to you as a cosmetologist, because they have a direct bearing on your well-being as well as on your clients' welfare. To protect individual and public health, every cosmetologist should know when, why, and how to use good sterilization and sanitation practices.

In order to understand the importance of sanitation and sterilization, a basic understanding of how *bacteria* (bak-**TEER**-ee-ah) affect our daily lives is most helpful.

BACTERIOLOGY

Bacteriology is the science that deals with the study of *microorganisms* (meye-kroh-**OR**-gah-niz-ems) called bacteria.

As a cosmetologist, you should understand how the spread of disease can be prevented and what precautions you must take to protect your health and your clients' health. Once you have an understanding of the relationship between bacteria and disease, you will understand the need for school and salon cleanliness and sanitation.

State boards of cosmetology and health departments require that a business that serves the public must follow certain sanitary precautions. Contagious diseases, skin infections, and blood poisoning are caused either by infectious bacteria being transmitted from one individual to another, or by the use of unsanitary implements (such as combs, brushes, hairpins, clippies, rollers, etc.). Dirty hands and fingernails are other sources of infectious bacteria.

Bacteria are minute, one-celled vegetable microorganisms found nearly everywhere. They are especially numerous in dust, dirt, refuse, and diseased tissues. Bacteria are also known as *germs* (**JURMS**) or *microbes* (**MEYE**-krohbs). Bacteria can exist almost anywhere: on the skin of the body, in water, air, decayed matter, secretions of body openings, on clothing, and beneath the nails.

Bacteria can be seen only with the aid of a *microscope* (**MEYE**-kroh-skohp). Fifteen hundred rod-shaped bacteria will barely cover the head of a pin.

TYPES OF BACTERIA

There are hundreds of different kinds of bacteria. However, bacteria are classified into two types, depending on whether they are beneficial or harmful.

1. Most bacteria are *nonpathogenic* (non-path-o-**JEN**-ik) organisms (helpful or harmless), which perform many useful functions, such as decomposing refuse and improving soil fertility. *Saprophytes* (**SAP**-ro-fights), nonpathogenic bacteria, live on dead matter and do not produce disease.
2. *Pathogenic* (path-o-**JEN**-ik) organisms (microbes or germs) are harmful, and although in the minority, produce disease when they invade plant or animal tissue. To this group belong the *parasites* (**PAR**-ah-sights), which require living matter for their growth.

It is because of pathogenic bacteria that beauty schools and salons must maintain certain sanitary and cleanliness standards.

Promo Power

SELLING PRODUCTS

It's important that you select items to sell in your salon with care. Your professional reputation is on the line when you endorse a product. A client won't purchase a product from you that she can buy at a discount store; clients purchase products from a salon professional because they believe them to be superior to consumer products—and because they trust you to sell them the product formulated for their type of hair.

The most successful way to build a booming retail business is to train your employees to start selling from the moment a client is left in their care. If that attitude prevails throughout the salon, the client will be conditioned to buy home maintenance products specifically for her type hair and skin.

Concentrate on an attractive visual presentation that is large and highly visible. When people can pick up and examine items it almost always results in sales. Frequently rotate and rearrange the items.

Everyone loves a bargain, so fill a special clearance basket with small items, tie a pretty bow on the basket, and make every item in the basket the same price. The profit will be less, but it will more than make up the loss by stimulating buyer interest.

Every item must have prices clearly marked. Most people dislike asking the price of anything.

—*From* Milady's Salon Solutions *by Louise Cotter*

PRONUNCIATIONS OF TERMS RELATING TO PATHOGENIC BACTERIA

Singular
coccus (**KOK**-us)
bacillus (bah-**SIL**-us)
spirillum (speye-**RIL**-um)
staphylococcus
 (staf-i-lo-**KOK**-us)
streptococcus
 (strep-to-**KOK**-us)
diplococcus
 (dip-lo-**KOK**-us)

Plural
cocci (**KOK**-si)
bacilli (ba-**SIL**-i)
spirilla (speye-**RIL**-a)
staphylococci
 (staf-i-lo-**KOK**-si)
streptococci
 (strep-to-**KOK**-si)
diplococci (dip-lo-**KOK**-si)

CLASSIFICATIONS OF PATHOGENIC BACTERIA

Bacteria have distinct shapes that help to identify them. Pathogenic bacteria are classified as follows (Fig. 2.1):

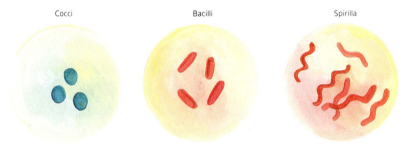

2.1—General forms of bacteria.

1. ***Cocci*** are round-shaped organisms that appear singly or in the following groups (Fig. 2.2):
   a) ***Staphylococci:*** Pus-forming organisms that grow in bunches or clusters. They cause abscesses, pustules, and boils.
   b) ***Streptococci:*** Pus-forming organisms that grow in chains. They cause infections such as strep throat.
   c) ***Diplococci:*** They grow in pairs and cause pneumonia.

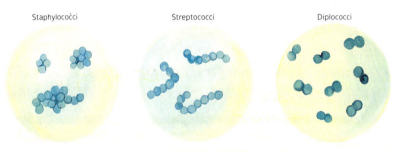

2.2—Groupings of bacteria.

2. *Bacilli* are short rod-shaped organisms. They are the most common bacteria and produce diseases such as tetanus (lockjaw), influenza, typhoid fever, tuberculosis, and diphtheria. (Fig. 2.3)
3. *Spirilla* are curved or corkscrew-shaped organisms. They are subdivided into several groups. Of chief importance to us is the *treponema pallida* (trep-o-**NE**-mah **PAL**-i-dah), which causes *syphilis* (**SIF**-i-lis).

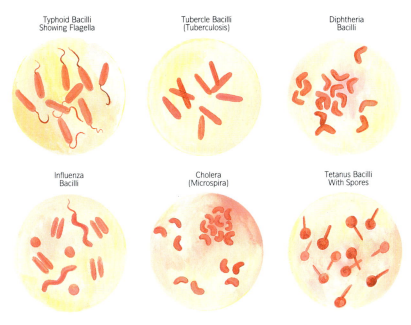

2.3—Disease-producing bacteria.

Movement of Bacteria

Cocci rarely show active *motility* (self-movement). They are transmitted on the air, in dust, or in the substance in which they settle. Bacilli and spirilla are both motile and use hairlike projections, known as *flagella* (flah-**JEL**-ah) or *cilia* (**SIL**-ee-a), to move about. A whiplike motion of these hairs propels bacteria about in liquid.

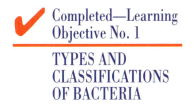

BACTERIAL GROWTH AND REPRODUCTION

Bacteria generally consist of an outer cell wall and internal *protoplasm* (**PROH**-toh-plaz-em), material needed to sustain life. They manufacture their own food from the surrounding environment, give off waste products, and grow and reproduce. Bacteria have two distinct phases in their life cycle: the *active* or *vegetative stage,* and the *inactive* or *spore-forming stage*.

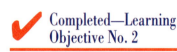

HOW BACTERIA GROW AND REPRODUCE

Active or Vegetative Stage

During the active stage, bacteria grow and reproduce. These microorganisms multiply best in warm, dark, damp, or dirty places where sufficient food is available.

When conditions are favorable, bacteria grow and reproduce. When they reach their largest size, they divide into two new cells. This division is called *mitosis*. The cells formed are called *daughter cells*. When conditions are unfavorable, bacteria die or become inactive. (See chapter on cells, anatomy, and physiology.)

Inactive or Spore-Forming Stage

Certain bacteria, such as the anthrax and tetanus bacilli, form *spherical spores* with tough outer coverings during their inactive stage. The purpose is to be able to withstand periods of famine, dryness, and unsuitable temperatures. In this stage, spores can be blown about and are not harmed by disinfectants, heat, or cold.

When favorable conditions are restored, the spores change into the active or vegetative form, then grow and reproduce.

BACTERIAL INFECTIONS

There can be no infection without the presence of pathogenic bacteria. An infection occurs when the body is unable to cope with the bacteria and their harmful toxins. A *local infection* is indicated by a boil or pimple that contains pus. The presence of *pus* is a sign of infection. Bacteria, waste matter, decayed tissue, body cells, and living and dead blood cells are all found in pus. Staphylococci are the most common pus-forming bacteria. A *general infection* results when the bloodstream carries the bacteria and their toxins to all parts of the body, as in syphilis.

A disease becomes *contagious* (kon-**TAY**-jus) or *communicable* (ko-**MYOO**-ni-kah-bil) when it spreads from one person to another by contact. Some of the more common contagious diseases that prevent a cosmetologist from working are tuberculosis, common cold, ringworm, scabies, head lice, and virus infections.

The chief sources of contagion are unclean hands and implements, open sores, pus, mouth and nose discharges, and the common use of drinking cups and towels. Uncovered coughing or sneezing and spitting in public also spread germs.

Pathogenic bacteria can enter the body through:

1. A break in the skin, such as a cut, pimple, or scratch.
2. The mouth (breathing or swallowing air, water, or food).
3. The nose (air).
4. The eyes or ears (dirt).

The body fights infection by means of:

1. Unbroken skin, which is the body's first line of defense.
2. Body secretions, such as perspiration and digestive juices.
3. White cells within the blood that destroy bacteria.
4. Antitoxins that counteract the toxins produced by bacteria.

Infections can be prevented and controlled through personal hygiene and public sanitation.

OTHER INFECTIOUS AGENTS

Filterable viruses (**FIL**-ter-a-bil **VEYE**-rus-es) are living organisms so small that they can pass through the pores of a porcelain filter. They cause the common cold and other respiratory (**RES**-pi-rah-torh-ee) and gastrointestinal (digestive tract) (gas-troh-in-**TES**-ti-nal) infections.

Parasites are organisms that live on other living organisms without giving anything in return.

Plant parasites or *fungi* (**FUN**-ji), such as molds, mildews, and yeasts, can produce contagious diseases, such as ringworm and *favus* (**FAY**-vus), a skin disease of the scalp.

Animal parasites are responsible for contagious diseases. For example, the itch mite burrows under the skin, causing *scabies* (**SKAY**-beez), and infection of the scalp by lice is called *pediculosis* (pe-dik-yoo-**LOH**-sis).

Contagious diseases caused by parasites should never be treated in a beauty school or salon. Clients should be referred to a physician.

IMMUNITY

Immunity (i-**MYOO**-ni-tee) is the ability of the body to destroy bacteria that have gained entrance, and thus to resist infection. Immunity against disease can be natural or acquired and is a sign of good health. *Natural immunity* means natural resistance to disease. It is partly inherited and partly developed through hygienic living. *Acquired immunity* is something the body develops after it has overcome a disease, or through inoculation.

A human disease carrier is a person who is personally immune to a disease yet can transmit germs to other people. *Typhoid* (**TEYE**-foid) *fever* and *diphtheria* (dif-**THEER**-i-a) can be transmitted in this manner.

Bacteria can be destroyed by disinfectants and by intense heat achieved by boiling, steaming, baking, or burning, and ultraviolet rays. (This subject is covered in the chapter on sterilization and sanitation.)

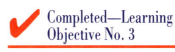

Completed—Learning Objective No. 3

THE RELATIONSHIP OF BACTERIA TO THE SPREAD OF DISEASE

ACQUIRED IMMUNE DEFICIENCY SYNDROME (AIDS)

Acquired immune deficiency syndrome (AIDS) is caused by the HIV virus. AIDS attacks and destroys the body's immune system. The disease may lie dormant in an infected person's system for up to ten years but can mature into a fatal disease in two to ten years.

Unlike most other viruses, HIV cannot be transferred through casual contact with an infected person, sneezing, or coughing. HIV is passed from one person to another through the transfer of bodily fluids such as semen and blood. The most common methods of transferring AIDS are sexual contact with an infected person, the use of or sharing of dirty hypodermic needles for intravenous drugs and the transfusion of infected blood. AIDS can also be transferred from mother to child during pregnancy and birth.

AIDS can be transferred in the salon through the use of unsanitized implements. If you cut a client infected with AIDS you might transfer blood to an implement. If you cut another client and transferred the AIDS-infected blood, that person might get AIDS.

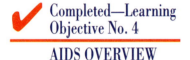

Completed—Learning Objective No. 4

AIDS OVERVIEW

REVIEW QUESTIONS

BACTERIOLOGY

1. Why is bacteriology necessary? *page 24*
2. Define bacteriology. *page 24*
3. What are bacteria? *page 24*
4. Where can bacteria exist? Give examples. *page 24*
5. Define two types of bacteria. *page 25*
6. What are parasites and saprophytes? *page 25*
7. Name and define three forms of bacteria. *page 26-27*
8. Name and define three types of cocci bacteria. *page 26*
9. How do bacteria multiply? *page 27*
10. Describe the active and inactive stages of bacteria. *page 27-28*
11. How does bacteria move about? *page 27*
12. Name two types of infection and define each. *page 28*
13. What is a contagious or communicable disease? *page 28*
14. How can infections be controlled or prevented? *page 29*
15. Name two diseases produced by a) plant parasites and b) animal parasites. *page 29*
16. Define immunity. Name two types. *page 29*
17. How can bacteria be destroyed? *page 29*

DECONTAMINATION AND INFECTION CONTROL

3

LEARNING OBJECTIVES

AFTER COMPLETING THIS CHAPTER, YOU SHOULD BE ABLE TO:

1. Explain and understand the importance of decontamination.
2. Explain the difference between sanitation, disinfection, and sterilization.
3. Discuss how to safely handle and use disinfectant products.
4. Describe which cleaners, equipment, and disinfectants are useful for salons.
5. Define universal sanitation and discuss your responsibilities as a salon professional.

INTRODUCTION

Clients love to see a clean salon. It gives them a feeling of confidence in both you and your special training. Clean and orderly salons make a positive statement. There is no better way to make a good first impression.

However, there is more to keeping the salon clean than sweeping the floor and vacuuming the rugs. If proper care is not taken you could contribute to the spread of diseases.

Controlling infection and disease is an important part of the salon industry. Clients depend upon you to ensure their safety. Protecting against the spread of infectious germs and other organisms is also required by federal and state regulations and for good reason. One careless action could cause injury or serious illness. Being a salon professional can be fun and rewarding, but it is also a great responsibility.

Disease-causing germs will be one of your biggest enemies in the salon. Fortunately, preventing the spread of dangerous diseases is easy, if you know how.

PREVENTION AND CONTROL

CONTAMINATION

Take a moment to look around you. What do you see? No matter where you are, you will always see a surface of some sort. The surface of the table, the wall, the floor, your hand…most things have a surface. No matter how clean these surfaces look, they are probably *contaminated*.

Surfaces of tools or other objects that are not free from dirt, oils, and microbes are contaminated. Any substance that causes contamination is called a *contaminant*. Many things can be contaminants. Hair in a comb or makeup on a towel are contaminants.

Tools and other surfaces in the salon can also be contaminated with bacteria, viruses, and fungi. Even tools that look clean are usually covered with these microorganisms.

DECONTAMINATION

It would be impossible to keep the salon free from all contamination, nor is it necessary to try. However, it is your responsibility as a salon professional to be on constant alert for disease-causing microorganisms.

Removing pathogens and other substances from tools or surfaces is called *decontamination*. There are three main levels of decontamination: sterilization, sanitation, and disinfection. However, only sanitation and disinfection are useful in the salon.

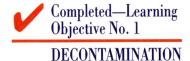

Completed—Learning Objective No. 1
DECONTAMINATION

STERILIZATION

Sterilization is the most effective type of decontamination against microbes. Sterilization completely destroys all living organisms on a surface. Sterilization even kills bacterial spores, the most resistant form of life on Earth.

The *steam autoclave*, the most popular method of physical sterilization and the most preferred due to its proven history of sterilizing, is like a pressure cooker. When steam is injected into a chamber at high pressure, it is possible to raise the temperature above that of boiling water. If something is left in the autoclave long enough, the high pressure and high heat will penetrate into all of the object's nooks and crannies. This will eventually kill all living organisms, including bacterial spores.

Another physical method of sterilization is the use of dry heat, a method more like an oven than a pressure cooker. Objects are placed into an ovenlike chamber and baked until all forms of life are dead.

Sterilization is the highest of the three levels of decontamination. It is a multi-step, time consuming, and difficult process. It is unnecessary, impractical, and virtually impossible to sterilize tools and surfaces in the salon.

Sterilization is used by dentists and surgeons. Their tools are designed to break and penetrate the skin barrier. For this reason, some estheticians feel it is important to sterilize needles and probes used to lance the skin. A simpler alternative would be to use disposable lancets or needles.

The word "sterilize" is often used incorrectly. For example, some practitioners tell clients that they are "sterilizing the nail plate or skin." This is impossible! Sterilizing the skin would quickly kill it and would destroy the nail plate, as well. In short, sterilization is impractical in salons.

SANITATION

The lowest level of decontamination is called *sanitation* or *sanitization*. These words are also frequently misused and misunderstood.

Sanitation means to "significantly reduce the number of pathogens found on a surface." Salon tools and other surfaces are sanitized by cleaning with soaps or detergents.

Sanitized surfaces may still harbor pathogens or other organisms. Removing hair from a brush and washing the brush with detergent is considered sanitation. Putting antiseptics on skin or washing your hands is another example of sanitation. Your hands may be very clean when you are finished, but they are covered with microorganisms found in the tap water and on the towel.

The Professional Look

Sanitation should be a part of everyone's normal routine. In this way, you and your co-workers can maintain a professional-look-

establishment. Following are some simple guidelines that will help keep the salon looking its best.

1. Floors should be swept clean whenever needed.
2. Hair, cotton balls, etc. should be picked up immediately.
3. Deposit all waste materials in a metal waste receptacle with a self-closing lid.
4. Mop floors and vacuum carpets daily.
5. It is important to control all types of dust.
6. Windows, screens, and curtains should be clean.
7. Regularly clean fans, ventilation systems, and humidifiers.
8. All work areas must be well lighted.
9. Salons need both hot and cold running water.
10. Rest rooms must be clean and tidy.
11. Remember to clean bathroom door handles.
12. Toilet tissue, paper towels, and pump-type antiseptic liquid soap must be provided.
13. Wash hands after using the rest room and between clients.
14. Clean sinks and drinking fountains regularly.
15. Separate or disposable drinking cups must be provided.
16. The salon must be free from insects and rodents.
17. Salons should never be used for cooking or living quarters.
18. Food must never be placed in refrigerators used to store salon products.
19. Eating, drinking, and smoking is prohibited in the salon.
20. Waste receptacles must be emptied regularly throughout the day.
21. Employees must wear clean, freshly washed clothing.
22. Always use freshly laundered towels on each client.
23. Capes or other covering should not contact client's skin.
24. Makeup, lipstick, puffs, pencils, and brushes must never be shared.
25. Clean cotton balls or sponges should be used to apply cosmetics and creams.
26. Remove products from containers with clean spatulas, not fingers.
27. All containers must be properly marked, tightly closed, and properly stored.
28. The outside of all containers should be kept clean.
29. Soiled or dirty linen are to be removed from the workplace and properly stored for cleaning.
30. Do not place any tools, combs, curlers, or bobby pins in your mouth or pockets.
31. Client gowns and headbands should be properly cleaned before being reused.
32. All tools and implements should be properly cleaned after each use and stored in a covered container.
33. Professionals should avoid touching their face, mouth, or eye area during services.
34. No pets or animals should ever be allowed in salons, except for trained Seeing Eye® dogs.

These are only a few of the things professionals must do in order to safeguard themselves and clients. Contact your local state board of cosmetology or health department for a complete list of regulations.

ANTISEPTICS

Antiseptics (an-ti-SEP-tiks) can kill bacteria or slow their growth, but they are not disinfectants. Antiseptics are weaker than disinfectants and are safe for application to skin. They are considered to be sanitizers and should never be used to replace disinfectants.

DISINFECTION

If sterilization is not practical and sanitation alone is not enough, what can you do to prevent the spread of dangerous organisms? Proper disinfection is the answer! *Disinfection* controls microorganisms on nonliving surfaces such as instruments and other implements. Disinfection is a higher level of decontamination than sanitation. It is second only to sterilization.

Disinfection is actually identical to sterilization, with one exception. Disinfection does not kill bacterial spores, but this is not necessary in the salon environment. It is important only in hospitals and other health care facilities.

Disinfectants are substances that kill microbes on contaminated tools and other nonliving surfaces. **Disinfectants are not for use on human skin, hair, or nails.** Never use disinfectants as hand cleaners. Any substance powerful enough to quickly and efficiently destroy pathogens can also damage skin. Always remember, disinfection products are serious, professional-strength tools. ✓

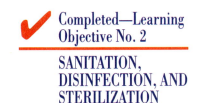

Completed—Learning Objective No. 2

SANITATION, DISINFECTION, AND STERILIZATION

READ BEFORE USING

Manufacturers take great care to develop safe and highly effective systems. However, being safe does not mean they cannot be dangerous. Any professional salon product can be dangerous if used incorrectly. Like all tools, disinfectants must always be used in strict accordance with manufacturer's instructions.

IMPORTANT INFORMATION

All disinfectants must be approved by the Environmental Protection Agency (EPA) and each individual state. The disinfectant's label must also have an *EPA registration number*. Look for this number when choosing a disinfectant. It is the only way to ensure that the product is both safe and effective.

Besides the EPA registration number, federal law requires manufacturers to give you other important information, such as directions for proper use, safety precautions, a list of active ingredients, and an important information sheet called a Material Safety Data Sheet (MSDS).

Take the time to read all of this vital information. Then you will be certain that you are protecting yourself and clients to the best of your ability!

> ### CAUTION
> *Disinfectants are too harsh for human skin or eye contact. Always wear gloves and safety glasses to prevent accidental exposure.*

OSHA

The Occupational Safety and Health Administration (OSHA) was created as part of the U.S. Department of Labor to regulate and enforce safety and health standards in the workplace. Regulating employee exposure to toxic substances and informing employees of the dangers of the materials used in the workplace are key functions of the Occupational Safety and Health Act of 1970. This act established the Hazard Communication Rule, which requires that chemical manufacturers and importers assess the hazards associated with their products. Material Safety Data Sheets and labeling are two important results of this law.

Material Safety Data Sheets provide all pertinent information on products, ranging from content and associated hazards, to combustion levels and storage requirements. These sheets should be available for every product used in the cosmetology school or salon, and may be obtained from the product's distributor. (Fig. 3.1)

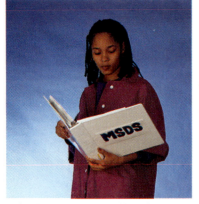

3.1—Read your Material Safety Data Sheets (MSDS).

The standards set by OSHA are important to the cosmetology industry because of the nature of the chemicals used, for instance, the mixing, storing, and disposal of chemicals; the general safety of the workplace; and, most important, the right of the cosmetologist to know what is contained in the products he or she uses.

HOSPITAL LEVEL DISINFECTANTS

The best way to learn to use disinfectants properly is to read the manufacturer's instructions. You should also periodically review these directions in case new information is added.

High quality disinfectants must perform several special jobs in the salon. They must be *bactericides* (bak-**TEER**-ih-sides) (kill harmful bacteria) and *fungicides* (**FUN**-jih-sides) (destroy fungus).

Disinfectants that perform both of these functions are called *hospital level disinfectants*. This is the level of disinfection that is ideal for the salon. Most hospital level disinfectants are also *viricides* (**VIR**-ih-sides) (kill viruses). It is recommended that tools and implements, except those which come in contact with blood or body fluids, be disinfected by complete immersion in an EPA registered, hospital level, bactericidal, virucidal and fungicidal disinfectant that is mixed and used according to the manufacturer's direction.

Some manufacturers have proven to the EPA that their disinfectants are effective against tuberculosis bacteria. These products are sold as *hospital level/tuberculocidal disinfectants*. It is recommended that tools and implements which have come in contact with blood or body fluids be disinfected by complete immersion in an EPA registered, hospital level/tuberculocidal disinfectant that is mixed and used according to the manufacturer's directions.

PROPER USE OF DISINFECTANTS

Even the best disinfectants won't work very well if used incorrectly. All implements should be thoroughly cleaned before soaking to avoid contaminating the disinfecting solution. Hair, nail filings, creams, oils, and makeup will lessen the effectiveness of the solution. Besides, a dirty jar of disinfectant wouldn't give your clients much confidence in your abilities.

Jars or containers used to disinfect implements are often incorrectly called *wet sanitizers*. Of course, the purpose of these containers is not to sanitize, but disinfect. The disinfecting soak solution must be changed daily unless otherwise directed by the manufacturer's instructions. (Fig. 3.2)

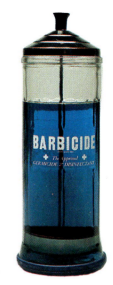

3.2—The disinfecting soak solution should be changed daily or according to manufacturer's instructions.

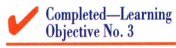

Completed—Learning Objective No. 3

USE AND SAFETY OF DISINFECTANT PRODUCTS

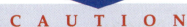

CAUTION
*Because blood can carry many pathogens, you should never touch a client's open sore or wound. Insist that clients with open sores (also known as **blood spills**) have a doctor certify they are not contagious. Be sure to properly clean and disinfect any implement that comes in contact with a cut or open sore in an EPA registered, hospital level/tuberculocidal disinfectant. Also, seal contaminated wipes or cotton balls in a plastic bag before disposing, then sanitize your hands.*

Promo Power

APPEARANCE CAN BE A SELLING POINT

Of course you're scrupulous about sanitizing and disinfecting in your salon. In an era when the public is more aware than ever of the spread of disease, practicing safety in the salon—whether it's a full-service salon, a nail salon, or a skincare salon—is absolutely essential.

But you can follow every rule about making your equipment and environment germfree, and it still may not be enough to convince your clients that your salon is "really clean." For the layperson with no training in sanitation, appearances are everything. The key is to make your salon *look* sparkling clean, even in areas where the danger of germs being spread is minimal. First impressions are always important and if a client walks in and sees dingy curtains or stained walls, the immediate thought will be, "This place is not clean."

Here is a checklist to make sure your first impression is a good one:
- Windows and drapes should be cleaned at least once a week.
- Doors should be clean and easy to open.
- Wall displays should be easy to clean and easy to change regularly.
- The reception desk should be neat and well organized.
- The reception area should contain ashtrays (if you allow smoking).
- Walls within the styling area should be easy to clean and freshly painted or covered.
- Rest rooms, mirrors, floors, and counter space around each work area should be kept clean.
- Floors should be made of a nonporous substance that is long wearing and easy to clean.
- The exterior of the salon should be well maintained and well lit.

TYPES OF DISINFECTANTS

QUATS

There are several types of salon disinfectants. ***Quaternary ammonium compounds (quats)*** (KWAH-ter-nah-ree ah-MOH-nee-um KOM-pownds [KWATS]) are one type. Quats are considered to be very safe and fast acting. Older formulas relied on only one quat and were not very effective. Newer products (called super quat formulas) use blends of several different quats that dramatically increase effectiveness.

Most quat solutions disinfect implements in 10 to 15 minutes. Leaving some tools in the solution for too long may damage them. Long-term exposure to any water solution or disinfectant may damage fine steel.

With today's modern formulas, corrosion of metal surfaces can be easily avoided, especially if you keep implements separated from each other while disinfecting. Metal implements such as scissors and nail clippers should be oiled regularly to keep them in perfect working order.

Quats are also very effective for cleaning table and counter tops.

PHENOLS

Like quats, *phenolic* (fee-**NOH**-lick) *disinfectants (phenols)* have been used for many years to disinfect implements. They too can be safe and extremely effective if used according to instructions. One disadvantage is that certain rubber and plastic materials may be softened or discolored by phenols.

Extra care should be taken to avoid skin contact with phenols. Phenolic disinfectants can cause skin irritation, and concentrated phenols can seriously burn the skin and eyes. Also, take care to keep phenols out of the reach of children as some are poisonous if accidentally ingested.

ALCOHOL, BLEACH, AND COMMERCIAL CLEANERS

The word *alcohol* is often misunderstood. Actually, there are thousands of types of alcohols. The three most common types are *methyl* (**METH**-il) *alcohol* (methanol), *ethyl* (**ETH**-il) *alcohol* (ethanol or grain alcohol), and *isopropyl* (eye-so-**PROH**-pil) *alcohol* (isopropanol or rubbing alcohol).

In the salon, ethyl and isopropyl alcohol are often used for disinfecting implements. To be effective, the strength of ethyl alcohol must be no less than 70%. Isopropyl alcohol's strength must be 99% or it is ineffective.

There are many disadvantages to using alcohols. They are extremely flammable, evaporate quickly, and are slow-acting, less-effective disinfectants. Alcohols corrode tools and cause sharp edges to become dull. The vapors formed upon evaporation can cause headaches and nausea in high concentrations or after prolonged exposure.

Household bleach (*sodium hypochlorite*) (**SOH**-dee-um high-poh-**KLOR**-ite) is an effective disinfectant, but shares some of the same drawbacks of alcohols. Neither bleach nor alcohols are professionally designed and tested for disinfection of salon implements. These may have been used extensively in the past, but have since been replaced by more advanced and effective technologies.

Although quats are perfectly suitable for cleaning any surface (unless otherwise specified in the manufacturer's directions), you may wish to clean floors, bathrooms, sinks, and waste receptacles with a commercial cleaner such as Lysol® or Pine-Sol®. Both are very effective disinfectants, but should not be used on salon implements. They are general, "household level" disinfectants and are not designed for professional tools.

ULTRASONIC CLEANERS

Ultrasonic baths or cleaners are useful when combined with disinfectants. Ultrasonic baths use high-frequency sound waves to create powerful, cleansing bubbles in the liquid. This cleansing action is an effective way to clean nooks and crannies that are impossible to reach with a brush. However, without an effective disinfectant solution, these devices will only sanitize implements.

Ultrasonic cleaners are a useful addition to your disinfection process, but are not required equipment. Many systems disinfect with great effectiveness without such devices. However, some feel this added cleaning benefit is well worth the extra expense.

DISINFECTANT SAFETY

Disinfectants are powerful, professional-strength tools that may be hazardous if used incorrectly. Some disinfectants are poisonous if ingested, and some can cause serious skin and eye damage, especially in a concentrated form.

A good rule to remember is: **Use Caution!** Wear gloves and safety glasses while mixing or using disinfectants. Always keep disinfectants away from children. (Fig. 3.3)

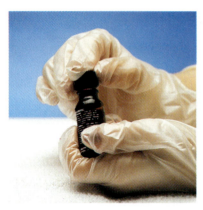

3.3—Wear gloves when using strong chemicals.

Use tongs or a draining basket to remove implements from disinfectants. Never pour alcohol, quats, phenols, or any other disinfectant over your hands. This foolish practice can cause skin disease and increase the chance of infection. Wash your hands with an antiseptic soap and dry them thoroughly.

Carefully weigh and measure all products to assure they perform at their peak efficiency. Never place any disinfectant or other product in an unmarked bottle. (Fig. 3.4)

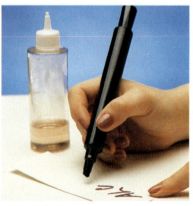

3.4—Label all containers. If the container isn't labeled, don't use it.

◆ CAUTION

*In the past, **formalin** was recommended as a disinfectant and fumigant in dry cabinet sanitizers. Although formalin is effective, **it is not safe for salon use**.*

*The gas released from formalin tablets or liquid is called **formaldehyde** (for-MAL-de-hide). Formaldehyde is a suspected human cancer causing agent. It is poisonous to inhale and is extremely irritating to the eyes, nose, throat, and lungs. It can also cause skin allergies, irritation, dryness, and rash.*

After long-term use, formaldehyde vapors can cause symptoms similar to chronic bronchitis or asthma. These symptoms usually worsen over time with continued exposure.

◆ **NOTE:** Avoid using bar soaps in the salon. Bar soap can actually grow bacteria. It is much more sanitary to provide pump-type liquid antiseptic soaps.

OTHER SURFACES

It is very important to properly disinfect combs, brushes, scissors, razors, nippers, electrodes, and other commonly used tools. But there are many other surfaces in the salon to consider. For example, table or counter tops, telephone receivers, door knobs, cabinet handles, mirrors, and cash registers. Any surface can be contaminated, especially if touched by clients and staff. These items must also be sanitized regularly.

Cosmetologists must also disinfect mixing utensils, combs, brushes, pins, clips, curlers, hair dryers, and chairs. Dirty fans and humidifiers can spread microbes throughout the salon. These devices should be properly cleaned on a regular basis.

Look around and you will see, there is far more to keeping the salon safe and sanitary than rinsing the sinks and wiping up spills.

◆ **NOTE:** To properly disinfect a surface, first clean with suitable cleaner, apply disinfectant, and leave wet for at least ten minutes. Wipe the surface dry. Reapply disinfectant and allow surface to air dry.

PROPER STORAGE OF IMPLEMENTS

Once tools are properly disinfected, they must be stored where they will remain free from contamination. Ultraviolet (UV) sanitizers are useful storage containers, however, they will not disinfect salon implements. Never use these devices to disinfect!

If you do not wish to use a UV cabinet, disinfected implements should be stored in a disinfected, dry and covered container.

ELECTRIC OR BEAD "STERILIZERS"

These devices do **not** sterilize implements. They can't even properly disinfect tools. They only give users a false sense of security.

To effectively sterilize an implement with dry heat, the tools must be heated to 325°F (approximately 163°C) for at least 30 minutes. Effective disinfection can only occur if the entire implement, including handle, is submerged. These type of devices are a dangerous gamble with your client's health. ✔

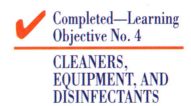

✔ Completed—Learning Objective No. 4

CLEANERS, EQUIPMENT, AND DISINFECTANTS

UNIVERSAL SANITATION

Protecting yourself and your clients requires you to do many things. You must use gloves and safety glasses, disinfectants and detergents, personal hygiene and salon cleanliness. When all of these things are performed together, it is called *universal sanitation*.

Universal sanitation must be a concerted effort. You must do all of these things in order to create a safe haven for your clients and co-workers.

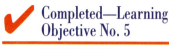

Completed—Learning Objective No. 5

UNIVERSAL SANITATION AND PROFESSIONAL RESPONSIBILITIES

YOUR PROFESSIONAL RESPONSIBILITY

You have many responsibilities as a salon professional. You have the responsibility to protect your clients from harm. You also have a responsibility to yourself. You must protect your health and safety, as well. Don't take short cuts when it comes to sanitation and disinfection. These important measures are designed to protect you, too!

Finally, you have a responsibility to your craft. When anyone acts unprofessionally in the salon, everyone's image is tarnished. Clients expect to see you act in a professional manner. This is how trust and respect are earned! ✔

REVIEW QUESTIONS

DECONTAMINATION AND INFECTION CONTROL

1. What is decontamination? page 32
2. Why is sterilization the most effective type of decontamination? page 33
3. Define sanitation and describe how salon tools and surfaces can be sanitized. page 33
4. What is the difference between an antiseptic and a disinfectant? page 35
5. What is the only way to ensure that a disinfectant is both safe and effective? page 35
6. What is an MSDS? page 36
7. List two qualities disinfectants must have to perform successfully in the salon. page 36
8. Name four types of salon disinfectants. page 38-39
9. Why is it recommended to avoid bar soaps in a salon? page 40
10. Why is formalin considered unsafe to use in the salon? page 40
11. What are the elements of universal sanitation? page 41

PROPERTIES OF THE SCALP AND HAIR

4

LEARNING OBJECTIVES

AFTER COMPLETING THIS CHAPTER, YOU SHOULD BE ABLE TO:

1. Explain the purpose of hair.
2. Define what hair is.
3. Define the chief composition of hair.
4. Define the divisions of hair.
5. Discuss the facts relating to hair structure, growth, and distribution.
6. Describe the theories pertaining to the life and replacement of hair.
7. List the causes of changes in hair color.
8. Know how to analyze a client's hair.
9. Define the disorders of hair.
10. Define basic scalp care.
11. Know how to perform scalp manipulation techniques.
12. Recognize the scalp and hair disorders commonly seen in the salon and school and know which can be treated there.

INTRODUCTION

As a hairstylist, it is important to have a technical knowledge of hair. This knowledge will be an asset to you as a professional cosmetologist.

Hair, like people, comes in a variety of colors, shapes, and sizes. To keep hair healthy and beautiful, proper attention must be given to its care and treatment. Applying a harsh cosmetic such as one that contains a lot of alcohol or providing improper hair services can cause the hair structure to become weakened or damaged. Knowledge and analysis of the client's hair, tactful suggestions for its improvement, and a sincere interest in maintaining its health and beauty should be primary concerns of every hairstylist.

HAIR

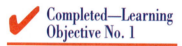

✔ **Completed—Learning Objective No. 1**

PURPOSE OF HAIR

The study of hair, technically called **trichology** (treye-KOL-o-jee), is important because stylists deal with hair on a daily basis. The chief purposes of hair are *adornment* and *protection* of the head from heat, cold, and injury. ✔

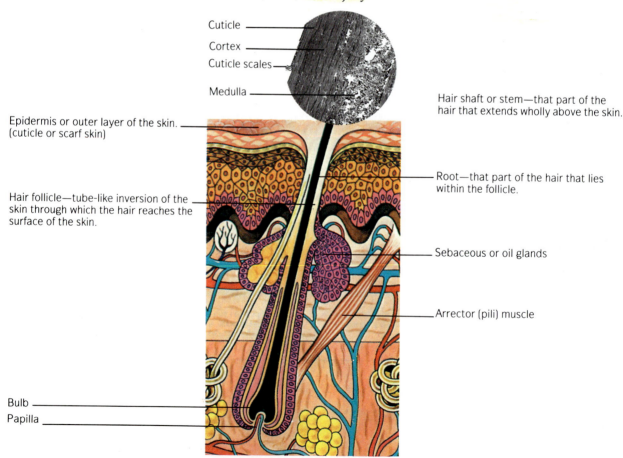

4.1—Cross section of skin and hair.

Hair is an *appendage* of the skin, a slender, threadlike outgrowth of the skin and scalp. (Fig. 4.1) There is no sense of feeling in hair, due to the absence of nerves.

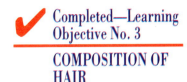

Completed—Learning Objective No. 2

DEFINITION OF HAIR

COMPOSITION OF THE HAIR

Hair is composed chiefly of the protein *keratin* (**KER**-ah-tin), which is found in all horny growths including the nails and skin. (Fig. 4.2) The chemical composition of hair varies with its color. Darker hair has more carbon and less oxygen; the reverse is true for lighter hair. Average hair is composed of 50.65% carbon, 6.36% hydrogen, 17.14% nitrogen, 5.0% sulfur, and 20.85% oxygen.

Completed—Learning Objective No. 3

COMPOSITION OF HAIR

DIVISIONS OF THE HAIR

Full-grown human hair is divided into two principal parts: the root and the shaft.

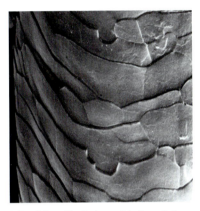

4.2—Magnified view of hair cuticle, which is composed of keratin.

1. The *hair root* is that portion of the hair structure located beneath the skin surface. This is the portion of the hair enclosed within the follicle.
2. The *hair shaft* is that portion of the hair structure extending above the skin surface.

Structures Associated with the Hair Root

The three main structures associated with the hair root are the follicle, bulb, and papilla.

The *follicle* (**FOL**-ih-kel) is a tubelike depression, or pocket, in the skin or scalp that encases the hair root. (Fig. 4.3) Each hair has its own follicle, which varies in depth depending on the thickness and location of the skin. (We talk later in this chapter about the different types of hair.) One or more oil glands are attached to each hair follicle.

The follicle does not run straight down into the skin or scalp, but is set at an angle so that the hair above the surface flows naturally

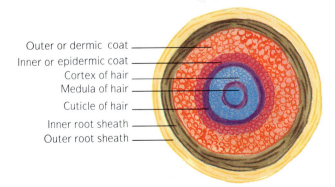

4.3—Cross section of the hair and follicle.

to one side. This natural flow is sometimes called the *hair stream* of the scalp. It is fascinating that nature has allowed for hair to emerge from the scalp slanting in a given direction.

The *bulb* is a thickened, club-shaped structure that forms the lower part of the hair root. The lower part of the hair bulb is hollowed out to fit over and cover the hair papilla.

The *papilla* (pa-**PIL**-ah) is a small, cone-shaped elevation located at the bottom of the hair follicle and fits into the hair bulb. Within the hair papilla is a rich blood and nerve supply that contributes to the growth and regeneration of the hair. It is through the papilla that nourishment reaches the hair bulb. As long as the papilla is healthy and well nourished, it produces hair cells that enable new hair to grow.

Structures Associated with Hair Follicles

The *arrector pili* (a-**REK**-tohr **PEYE**-leye) is a small involuntary muscle attached to the underside of a hair follicle. Fear or cold causes it to contract and the hair stands up straight, giving the skin the appearance of "gooseflesh." Eyelash and eyebrow hair do not have arrector pili muscles.

Sebaceous (si-**BAY**-shus), or oil, glands consist of little sac-like structures in the dermis. Their ducts are connected to hair follicles. Sebaceous glands frequently become troublemakers by overproducing and bringing on a common form of oily dandruff. Normal secretion of an oily substance from these glands, called *sebum* (**SEE**-bum), gives luster and pliability to the hair and keeps the skin surface soft and supple. The production of sebum is influenced by diet, blood circulation, emotional disturbances, stimulation of endocrine glands, and drugs.

Diet influences the general health of the hair. Eating too much sweet, starchy, and fatty foods can cause the sebaceous glands to become overactive and secrete too much sebum.

Blood circulation. The hair derives its nourishment from the blood supply, which, in turn, depends on the foods we eat for certain elements. In the absence of necessary foods, the health of the hair can be affected.

Emotional disturbances are linked with the health of the hair through the nervous system. Unhealthy hair can be an indication of an unhealthy emotional state.

Endocrine glands. The secretions of the endocrine glands influence the health of the body. Any disturbance of these glands can affect the health of the body and, ultimately, the health of the hair.

Drugs, such as hormones, can adversely affect the hair's ability to receive permanent waving and other chemical services. ✓

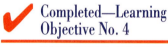

Completed—Learning Objective No. 4

DIVISIONS OF THE HAIR

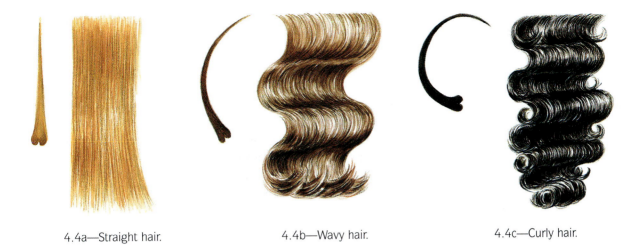

4.4a—Straight hair.   4.4b—Wavy hair.   4.4c—Curly hair.

HAIR SHAPES

Hair usually has one of three general shapes. (See Figs. 4.4a–c) As it grows out, hair assumes the shape, size, and curve of the follicle. A cross-sectional view of the hair under the microscope reveals that:

1. Straight hair is usually round.
2. Wavy hair is usually oval.
3. Curly or kinky hair is almost flat.

There is no strict rule regarding cross-sectional shapes of hair. Oval, straight, and curly hair have been found in all shapes. A myth exists that race or nationality determines the shape of hair—this is false. Anyone can have straight, wavy, or curly hair no matter what race or nationality. The direction of a hair as it projects out of the follicle determines each person's hair shape.

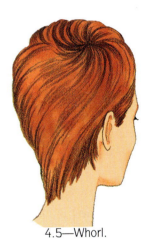

4.5—Whorl.

Direction of Hair Growth

Hair stream. Hair flowing in the same direction is known as the hair stream. It is the result of the follicles sloping in the same direction. Two such streams, sloping in opposite directions, form a natural parting of the hair.

Whorl. Hair that forms a circular pattern, as in the crown, is called a whorl. (Fig. 4.5)

Cowlick. A tuft of hair standing up is known as a cowlick. Cowlicks are more noticeable at the front hairline. However, they may be located on other parts of the scalp. When shaping or styling the hair, it is important to consider the direction of cowlicks. (Fig. 4.6)

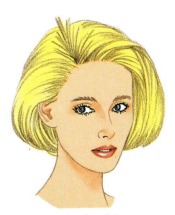

4.6—Cowlick.

LAYERS OF THE HAIR

The structure of the hair is composed of cells arranged in three layers (Also see Fig. 4.3 on page 45):

1. *Cuticle* (**KYOO**-ti-kel). The outside horny layer is composed of transparent, overlapping, protective scalelike cells, pointing away from the scalp toward the hair ends. Chemicals raise these scales so that solutions such as chemical relaxers, hair color, or permanent wave solutions can enter the hair cortex. The cuticle protects the inner structure of the hair.
2. *Cortex* (**KOR**-teks). The middle or inner layer, which gives strength and elasticity to the hair, is made up of a fibrous substance formed by elongated cells. This layer contains the pigment that gives the hair its color.
3. *Medulla* (mi-**DUL**-ah). The innermost layer is referred to as the pith, or marrow, of the hair shaft and is composed of round cells. The medulla may be absent in fine and very fine hair.

HAIR DISTRIBUTION

Hair is distributed all over the body, except on the palms of the hands, soles of the feet, lips, and eyelids. There are three types of hair on the body:

1. *Long hair* protects the scalp against the sun's rays and injury, gives adornment to the head, and forms a pleasing frame for the face. Soft, long hair also grows in the armpits of both sexes and on the faces of men. Male hormones, however, make a man's facial hair coarser than a woman's.
2. *Short or bristly hair*, such as the eyebrows and eyelashes, adds beauty and color to the face. Eyebrows divert sweat from the eyes. The eyelashes help protect the eyes from dust particles and light glare.
3. *Lanugo* (lah-**NOO**-goh) hair is the fine, soft, downy hair on the cheeks, forehead, and nearly all other areas of the body. It helps in the efficient evaporation of perspiration.

Technical Terms Given to Hair on the Head and Face

Barba (**BAR**-ba)—the face
Capilli (kah-**PIL**-i)—the head
Cilia (**SIL**-ee-a)—the eyelashes
Supercilia (soo-per-**SIL**-ee-a)—the eyebrows (Fig. 4.7)

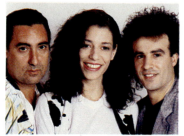

4.7—Hair on the head and face.

CHAPTER 4 PROPERTIES OF THE SCALP AND HAIR ◆ 49

HAIR GROWTH

If the hair is normal and healthy, each individual hair goes through a steady *cycle* of events: ***growth, fall,*** and ***replacement.*** You will notice that the average growth of healthy hair on the scalp is about ½″ (1.25 cm) per month. The rate of growth of human hair differs on specific parts of the body, between sexes, among races, and with age. Scalp hair also differs among individuals in strength, elasticity, and waviness.

The growth of scalp hair occurs more rapidly between the ages of 15 to 30, but declines sharply between 50 to 60. Scalp hair grows faster on women than on men. Hair growth also is influenced by seasons of the year, nutrition, health, and hormones.

Climatic conditions and *seasonal changes* affect hair in the following ways:

1. Humidity and moisture deepen the natural wave.
2. Cold air causes the hair to contract.
3. Heat causes the hair to swell or expand and absorb moisture.

Here are some myths about hair growth:

1. Close clipping, shaving, trimming, cutting, or singeing have an effect on the rate of hair growth. This is *not* true.
2. The application of ointments and oils increases hair growth. This is *not* true. Ointments and oils lubricate the hair shaft, but they *do not* feed the hair.
3. Hair grows after death. This is *not* true. The flesh and skin contract, thus there is the appearance of hair growth.
4. Singeing the hair seals in the natural oil. This is *not* true.

Normal Hair Shedding

A certain amount of hair is shed daily. This is nature's method of making way for new hair. The average daily shedding is estimated at 75 to 150 hairs. Hair loss beyond this estimated average indicates some scalp or hair abnormality.

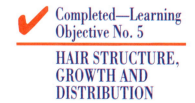

Completed—Learning Objective No. 5

HAIR STRUCTURE, GROWTH AND DISTRIBUTION

LIFE AND DENSITY OF THE HAIR

The exact life span of hair has not been agreed upon. The average life of hair ranges from 4 to 7 years. Factors such as sex, age, type of hair, heredity, and health have a bearing on the duration of hair life.

The area of an average head is about 120 square inches (780 cm^2). There is an average of 1,000 hairs to a square inch (6.5 cm^2). The number of hairs on the head varies with the color of the hair: blonde, 140,000; brown, 110,000; black, 108,000; red, 90,000.

NATURAL REPLACEMENT OF THE HAIR

Hair depends on the papilla for its growth. As long as the papilla is not destroyed, the hair will grow. If the hair is pulled out from the roots, it will grow again. But should the papilla be destroyed, the hair will never grow again. In humans, new hair replaces old hair in the following manner:

1. The bulb loosens and separates from the papilla. (Fig. 4.8a)
2. The bulb moves upward in the follicle.
3. The hair moves slowly to the surface where it is shed.
4. The new hair is formed by cell division, which takes place at the root of the hair around the papilla. (Fig. 4.8b)

✓ **Completed—Learning Objective No. 6**

LIFE AND REPLACEMENT OF THE HAIR

Eyebrows and eyelashes are replaced every 4 to 5 months.

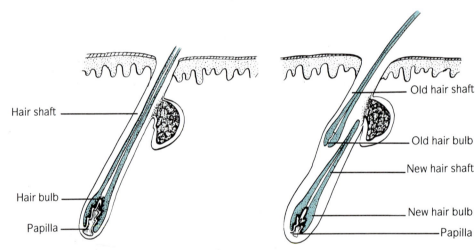

4.8a—At an early stage of shedding, the hair shows its separation from the papilla.

4.8b—At a later stage of the hair shedding, you will note a new hair growing from the same papilla.

COLOR OF THE HAIR

The natural color of hair, its strength, and its texture depend mainly on heredity. The cortex contains coloring matter, minute grains of *melanin* (**MEL**-a-nin), or pigment. Although there is no definite scientific proof, it appears that pigment is derived from the color-forming substances in the blood, as is all pigment of the human body. The color of a person's hair, how light or dark it is, depends on the number of grains of pigment in each strand.

An *albino* (al-**BEYE**-no) is a person born with white hair, the result of an absence of coloring matter in the hair shaft, accompanied by no marked pigment coloring in the skin or irises of the eyes.

To give successful hair lightening and tinting services, you need to know about natural hair color and distribution of hair pigment.

Graying of Hair

Gray hair is caused by the absence of color pigment in the cortical layer. It is really *mottled* hair—spots of white or whitish yellow scattered about in the hair shafts. Gray hair is just that—it grows that way from the hair bulb. It does not begin to grow as another color that turns gray.

In most cases, the graying of hair is a result of the natural aging process in humans, although graying also can occur as a result of some serious illness or nervous shock. An early diminishing of pigment brought on by emotional tensions can also cause the hair to turn gray.

Premature graying of hair in a young person is usually the result of a defect in pigment formation occurring at birth. Often it will be found that several members of a family are affected with premature grayness.

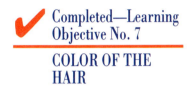

Completed—Learning Objective No. 7

COLOR OF THE HAIR

Question & Answer

CONDITIONING

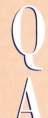

Many clients feel that conditioners do nothing but soften the hair. How can I promote conditioners other than creme rinses?

You may know the value of hair-conditioning treatments, but unless you convey that information to your clients they may not have the same faith in the service as you.

How about having a little brochure printed to let your clients know exactly why you suggest conditioners to those with less than healthy hair? The brochure could contain facts pertaining to different types of conditioners and their functions, beneficial ingredients, which treatment is recommended for what hair condition, the price of treatments and ingredients listed in layperson's terminology so the client can understand exactly what she or he is getting.

It's surprising to note that "conditioning" services for the hair and scalp consistently remain in a high position when compared to other salon services. These services seldom fall below fourth place in number of salon services and rank as high as seventh in dollar volume. Does that surprise you? It shouldn't, considering that women spend more than $500 million dollars annually on conditioning services alone.

Conditioners are meant to restore damaged or dry hair to lustrous health. They are formulated to restore moisture, replenish protein, add strength, soften the hair, close frayed cuticle, add luster, cause the hair to look thicker, and remove tangles.

The best and most ethical policy for the sale and use of any hair-care product (including conditioners) is to properly analyze the problem and use only that product that will correct the problem.

—*From* Milady's Salon Solutions *by Louise Cotter*

HAIR ANALYSIS

Much of the cosmetologist's time is taken up with servicing and styling clients' hair. For this reason, you should be able to recognize the condition and type of a client's hair and be able to analyze it.

CONDITION OF THE HAIR

Knowledge of hair and skill in determining its condition can be acquired by constant observation using the senses available to you: sight, touch, hearing, and smell.

1. *Sight*. Observing the hair will immediately give you some knowledge about its condition. Being able to look at hair contributes approximately 15% to its analysis, and touching the hair is the final determining factor.
2. *Touch*. Cosmetologists are guided by the touch or feel of the hair in making a professional hair analysis. When the sense of touch is fully developed, fewer mistakes will be made in judging the hair.
3. *Hearing*. Listen to what clients tell you about their hair, health problems, reactions to cosmetics and medications they might be taking. You will be in a better position to analyze the condition of hair more accurately.
4. *Smell*. Unclean hair and certain scalp disorders create an odor. If the client generally has good health, you might suggest regular shampooing and proper rinsing.

QUALITIES OF THE HAIR

Qualities by which human hair is analyzed are *texture*, *porosity*, and *elasticity*.

Texture

Hair texture refers to the degree of coarseness or fineness of the hair, which may vary on different parts of the head. Variations in hair texture are due to:

1. *Diameter of the hair*, whether coarse, medium, fine, or very fine. Coarse hair has the greatest diameter; very fine hair has the smallest.
2. *Feel of the hair*, whether harsh, soft, or wiry.

Medium hair is the normal type most commonly seen in the salon or school. This type of hair does not present any special problem. *Fine* or *very fine hair* requires special care. Its microscopic structure usually reveals that only two layers, the cortex and cuticle, are present. *Wiry hair*, whether coarse, medium, or fine, has a hard, glassy finish caused by the cuticle scales lying flat against the hair shaft. It takes longer for chemicals such as permanent wave solutions, tints, or lighteners to penetrate this type of hair.

Porosity

Hair porosity is the ability of all types of hair to absorb moisture *(hygroscopic quality)*. Hair has *good porosity* when the cuticle layer is raised from the hair shaft and can absorb a fair or normal amount of moisture or chemicals. *Moderate porosity* (normal hair) is most often seen in the salon or school. It is less porous than hair with good porosity. Usually hair with good or moderate porosity presents no problem when receiving hair services, whether permanent waving, hair tinting, or lightening. *Poor porosity* (resistant hair) exists when the cuticle layer is lying close to the hair shaft and absorbs the least amount of moisture. Hair with poor porosity requires thorough analysis and strand tests before the application of hair cosmetics. *Extreme porosity* is seen in hair in poor condition. It may be due to tinting, lightening, or damage from continuous or faulty treatments.

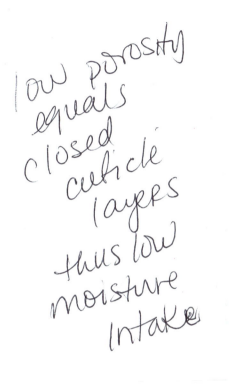

Elasticity

Hair elasticity is the ability of hair to stretch and return to its original form without breaking. Hair can be classified as having good elasticity, normal elasticity, or poor elasticity. (Refer to the chapter on permanent waving for more information.) Hair with normal elasticity is springy and has a lively and lustrous appearance. Normal dry hair is capable of being stretched about one-fifth of its length; it springs back when released. Wet hair can be stretched 40% to 50% of its length. Porous hair stretches more than hair with poor porosity.

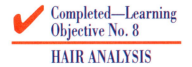

Completed—Learning Objective No. 8

HAIR ANALYSIS

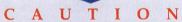

CAUTION

You should see by now that hair is complex and you must analyze each client individually. Never make a snap judgment based on race or nationality that a client will have a particular hair type.

DISORDERS OF THE HAIR

CANITIES

Canities (ka-**NIT**-eez) is the technical term for gray hair. Its immediate cause is the loss of natural pigment in the hair. There are two types:

1. Congenital canities exists at or before birth. It occurs in albinos and occasionally in persons with normal hair. A patchy type of congenital canities may develop either slowly or rapidly, depending upon the cause of the condition.

2. Acquired canities may be due to old age, or onset may occur prematurely in early adult life. Causes of acquired canities may be worry, anxiety, nervous strain, prolonged illness, or heredity.

RINGED HAIR

Ringed hair is alternate bands of gray and dark hair.

HYPERTRICHOSIS

Hypertrichosis (hi-per-tri-**KOH**-sis), or *hirsuties*, means superfluous hair, an abnormal development of hair on areas of the body normally bearing only downy hair. *Treatment:* Tweeze or remove by depilatories, electrolysis, shaving, or epilation.

TRICHOPTILOSIS

Trichoptilosis (tri-kop-ti-**LOH**-sis) is the technical term for *split hair ends*. (Fig. 4.9a) *Treatment:* The hair should be well oiled to soften and lubricate the dry ends. The ends also may be removed by cutting.

TRICHORRHEXIS NODOSA

Trichorrhexis nodosa (**TRIK**-o-rek-sis no-**DO**-sa), or *knotted hair*, is a dry, brittle condition including formation of nodular swellings along the hair shaft. (Fig. 4.9b) The hair breaks easily and there is a brush-like spreading out of the fibers of the broken-off hair along the hair shaft. Softening the hair with conditioners may prove beneficial.

MONILETHRIX

Monilethrix (moh-**NIL**-e-thriks) is the technical term for *beaded hair*. (Fig. 4.9c) The hair breaks between the beads or nodes. Scalp and hair treatments may improve the hair condition.

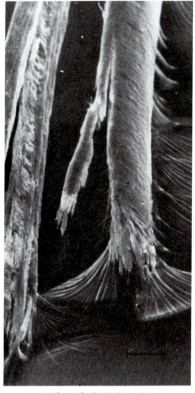 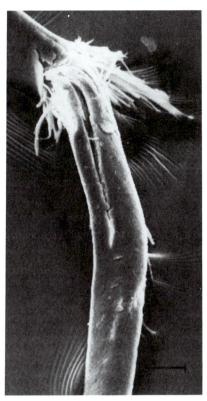 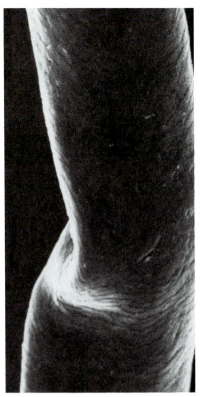

4.9a—Split hair ends.   4.9b—Knotted hair.   4.9c—Beaded hair.

FRAGILITAS CRINIUM

Fragilitas crinium (frah-**JIL**-i-tas **KRI**-nee-um) is the technical term for **brittle hair** or split ends. The hairs may split at any part of their length. Conditioning hair treatments may be recommended. ✔

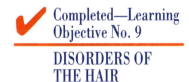

SCALP CARE

A basic requisite for a healthy scalp is cleanliness and stimulation. The scalp and hair should be kept clean by frequent treatment and shampooing. A healthy, clean scalp will resist a variety of disorders. ✔

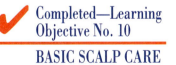

SCALP MANIPULATIONS

Since the same manipulations are given with all scalp treatments, you should learn to give them with a continuous, even motion, which will stimulate the scalp and/or soothe the client's tension. Scalp massage is most effectively applied as a series of treatments, once a week for normal scalp and more frequently for scalp disorders, under the direction of a dermatologist.

Anatomy

Knowing the muscles, the location of blood vessels, and the nerve points of the scalp and neck will help guide you to those areas in which massage movements are to be directed for the most beneficial results. (See chapter on cells, anatomy, and physiology.)

Scalp Manipulation Technique

There are several ways in which scalp manipulations may be given. The following routine may be changed to meet your instructor's requirements.

With each massage movement, place the hands under the hair so the length of the fingers, balls of the fingertips, and cushions of the palms can stimulate the muscles, nerves, and blood vessels of the scalp area.

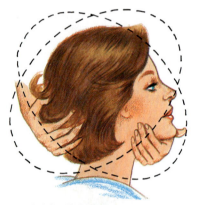

4.10—Relaxing movement.

1. RELAXING MOVEMENT. Cup the client's chin in your left hand; place your right hand at the base of her skull, and rotate head gently. Reverse positions of your hands and repeat. (See Fig. 4.10)

2. SLIDING MOVEMENT. Place your fingertips on each side of the client's head; slide your hands firmly upward, spreading the fingertips until they meet at the top of the head. Repeat four times. (See Fig. 4.11)

3. SLIDING AND ROTATING MOVEMENT. Same as movement No. 2, except that after sliding the fingertips 1" (2.5 cm), you rotate and move the client's scalp. Repeat four times. (See Fig. 4.12)

4. FOREHEAD MOVEMENT. Hold the back of the client's head with your left hand. Place stretched thumb and fingers of your right hand on the client's forehead. Move your hand slowly and firmly upward to 1" (2.5 cm) past the hairline. Repeat four times. (See Fig. 4.13)

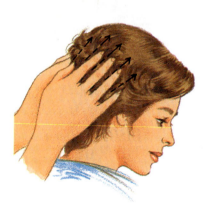

4.11—Sliding movement.

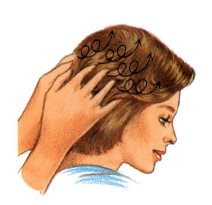

4.12—Sliding and rotating movement.

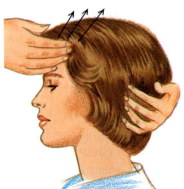

4.13—Forehead movement.

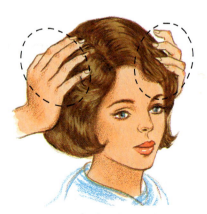

4.14—Scalp movement.

CHAPTER 4   PROPERTIES OF THE SCALP AND HAIR ◆ 57

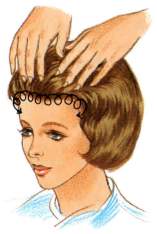

4.15—Hairline movement.

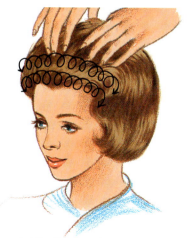

4.16—Front scalp movement.

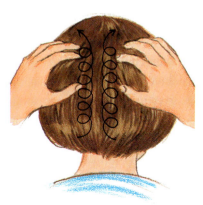

4.17—Back scalp movement.

5. SCALP MOVEMENT. Place the palms of your hands firmly against the client's scalp. Lift the scalp in a rotary movement, first with your hands placed above her ears, and second with your hands placed at the front and back of her head. (See Fig. 4.14)

6. HAIRLINE MOVEMENT. Place the fingers of both hands at the client's forehead. Massage around her hairline by lifting and rotating. (See Fig. 4.15)

7. FRONT SCALP MOVEMENT. Dropping back 1" (2.5 cm), repeat preceding movement over entire front and top of the scalp. (See Fig. 4.16)

8. BACK SCALP MOVEMENT. Place the fingers of each hand on the sides of the client's head. Starting below her ears, manipulate the scalp with your thumbs, working upward to the crown. Repeat four times. Repeat thumb manipulations, working toward the center back of the head. (See Fig. 4.17)

9. EAR-TO-EAR MOVEMENT. Place your left hand on the client's forehead. Massage from the right ear to the left ear along the base of her skull with the heel of your hand, using a rotary movement. (See Fig. 4.18)

10. BACK MOVEMENT. Place your left hand on the client's forehead and stand to the left of her. Using your right hand, rotate from the base of the client's neck, along the shoulder, and back across the shoulder blade to the spine. Slide your hand up the client's spine to the base of her neck. Repeat on the opposite side. (See Fig. 4.19)

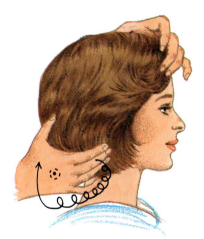

4.18—Ear-to-ear movement.

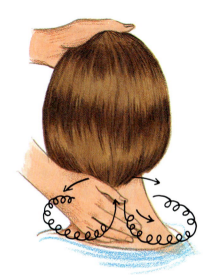

4.19—Back movement.

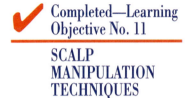

✓ Completed—Learning Objective No. 11

SCALP MANIPULATION TECHNIQUES

11. SHOULDER MOVEMENT. Place both your palms together at the base of the client's neck. With rotary movement, catch muscles in the palms and massage along the shoulder blades to the point of her shoulders, and then back again. Then massage from the shoulders to the spine and back again. (See Fig. 4.20)

12. SPINE MOVEMENT. Massage from the base of the client's skull down the spine with a rotary movement. Using a firm finger pressure, bring your hand slowly to the base of the client's skull. (See Fig. 4.21) ✔

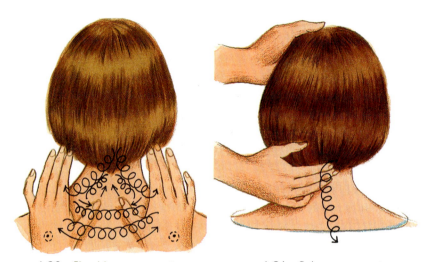

4.20—Shoulder movement.   4.21—Spine movement.

DISORDERS OF THE SCALP

Just as the skin is continually being shed and replaced, the uppermost layer of the scalp is also being cast off all the time. Ordinarily, these **horny scales** loosen and fall off freely. The natural shedding of these horny scales should not be mistaken for dandruff.

DANDRUFF

Dandruff consists of small, white scales that usually appear on the scalp and hair. The medical term for dandruff is ***pityriasis*** (pit-i-**REYE**-ah-sis). Long neglected, excessive dandruff can lead to baldness. The nature of dandruff is not clearly defined by medical authorities although it is generally believed to be of infectious origin. Some authorities hold that it is due to a specific microbe.

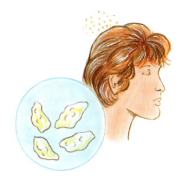 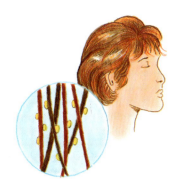

4.22a—Pityriasis capitis simplex.   4.22b—Pityriasis steatoides.

A direct cause of dandruff is the excessive shedding of the *epithelial,* or surface, *cells.* Instead of growing to the surface and falling off, these horny scales accumulate on the scalp.

Indirect or associated causes of dandruff are a sluggish condition of the scalp, possibly due to poor circulation, infection, injury, lack of nerve stimulation, improper diet, and uncleanliness. Contributing causes are the use of strong shampoos and insufficient rinsing of the hair after a shampoo. The two principal types of dandruff are:

1. *Pityriasis capitis simplex* (kah-**PEYE**-tis **SIM**-pleks)—dry type. (Fig. 4.22a)
2. *Pityriasis steatoides* (ste-a-**TOY**-dez)—a greasy or waxy type. (Fig. 4.22b)

Pityriasis capitis simplex (dry dandruff) is characterized by an itchy scalp and small white scales, which are usually attached to the scalp in masses, or scattered loosely in the hair. Occasionally, they are so profuse that they fall to the shoulders. Dry dandruff is often the result of a sluggish scalp caused by poor circulation, lack of nerve stimulation, improper diet, emotional and glandular disturbances, or uncleanliness. *Treatment:* Frequent scalp treatments, use of mild shampoos, regular scalp massage, daily use of antiseptic scalp lotions, and applications of scalp ointments.

Pityriasis steatoides (greasy or waxy type of dandruff) is a scaly condition of the epidermis (surface skin). The scales become mixed with sebum, causing them to stick to the scalp in patches. There may be itchiness, causing the person to scratch the scalp. If the greasy scales are torn off, bleeding or oozing of sebum may follow. Medical treatment is advisable.

Both forms of dandruff are considered to be contagious and can be spread by the common use of brushes, combs, and other articles. Therefore, the cosmetologist must take the necessary precautions to sanitize everything that comes into contact with the client.

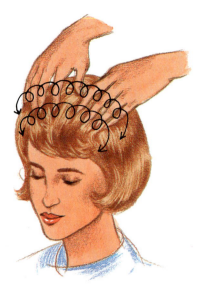

4.23a—Applying indirect high-frequency current, cosmetologist manipulates the scalp.

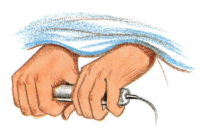

4.23b—While cosmetologist manipulates the scalp, the client holds metal electrode.

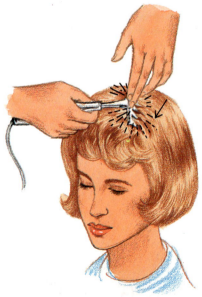

4.23c—Applying high-frequency current with glass rake electrode.

Dandruff Treatment

A scalp with a dandruff condition may be treated by using the following procedure:

1. Drape client. (See chapter on draping.)
2. Brush the client's hair for 5 minutes.
3. Apply a scalp preparation according to the scalp's condition (dry or oily). (See sections on dry and oily hair scalp treatments on pages 64 and 65.)
4. Apply infrared lamp for about 5 minutes. (See chapter on electricity and light therapy.)
5. Give scalp manipulations, using indirect high-frequency current. (Figs. 4.23a, 4.23b) (See chapter on electricity and light therapy.)
6. Shampoo with corrective anti-dandruff lotion.
7. Thoroughly towel-dry the hair.
8. Use direct high-frequency current for 3 to 5 minutes. (Fig. 4.23c) (See chapter on electricity and light therapy.)
9. Apply scalp preparation suitable for the condition.
10. Set, dry, and style the hair.
11. Clean up your workstation.

ALOPECIA

Alopecia (al-oh-**PEE**-shee-ah) is the technical term for any abnormal hair loss. The natural falling out of the hair should not be confused with alopecia. As we learned earlier, when hair has grown to its full length, it falls out and is replaced by a new hair. The natural shedding of hair occurs most frequently in spring and fall. Hair loss due to alopecia is not replaced unless special treatments are given to encourage hair growth. Hairstyles such as ponytails and tight braids cause tension on the hair and can contribute to constant hair loss or baldness.

Alopecia senilis (se-**NIL**-is) is the form of baldness that occurs in old age. This loss of hair is permanent.

Alopecia prematura (pre-mah-**CHUR**-ah) is the form of baldness that begins any time before middle age with a slow, thinning process. This condition is caused when hairs fall out and are replaced by weaker ones.

Alopecia areata (air-ee-**AH**-tah) is the sudden falling out of hair in round patches, or baldness in spots, sometimes caused by anemia, scarlet fever, typhoid fever, or syphilis. Patches are round or irregular in shape and can vary in size from ½" to 2" or 3" (1.3 to 5.1 or 7.6 cm) in diameter. Affected areas are slightly depressed, smooth, and very pale, due to a decreased blood supply. In most conditions of

CHAPTER 4   PROPERTIES OF THE SCALP AND HAIR ◆ 61

alopecia areata, the nervous system has been subjected to some injury. Since the flow of blood is influenced by the nervous system, the affected area also is poorly nourished. (Fig. 4.24)

Treatment for Alopecia
Alopecia appears in a variety of different forms, caused by many abnormal conditions. Sometimes an alopecia condition can be improved by proper scalp treatments.

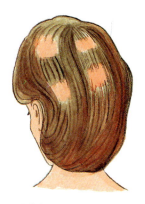

4.24—Alopecia areata.

Procedure for Alopecia Treatment
1. Drape client.
2. Brush the client's hair for about 5 minutes.
3. Apply a medicated scalp ointment as directed by a physician.
4. Apply infrared light for about 5 minutes.
5. Give scalp manipulations. You may use the faradic or indirect high-frequency current.
6. Use a mild shampoo.
7. Towel-dry the hair.
8. Apply direct high-frequency current for about 5 minutes.
9. Apply medicated scalp lotion.
10. Repeat scalp manipulations; include neck, shoulders, and upper back.
11. Set hair; dry with warm or cool air, and style hair.
12. Clean up your workstation.

Procedure for Alopecia Areata Treatment
1. Drape client.
2. Give regular scalp manipulations.
3. Shampoo the hair according to its condition; if scalp is very tender, use a mild shampoo.
4. Dry the hair and scalp thoroughly.
5. Expose the scalp to ultraviolet rays for 5 to 10 minutes, especially the bald spots. (Fig. 4.25)
6. Apply ointment or lotion with light manipulations on the bald spots.
7. Apply high-frequency current for about 5 minutes. If an ointment is used, apply direct current; if a lotion is used, apply indirect current.
8. Style the hair, using a comb only.
9. Clean up your workstation.

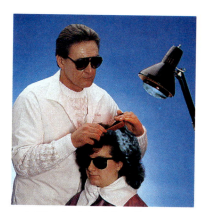

4.25—Applying ultraviolet rays.

VEGETABLE PARASITIC INFECTIONS

Tinea (**TIN**-ee-ah) is the medical term for ringworm. Ringworm is caused by vegetable parasites. All forms are contagious and can be transmitted from one person to another. The disease is commonly carried by scales or hairs containing fungi. Bathtubs, swimming pools, and unsanitized articles are also sources of transmission.

Ringworm starts with a small, reddened patch of little blisters. Several such patches may be present. Any ringworm condition should be referred to a physician.

Tinea capitis (kah-**PEYE**-tis), ringworm of the scalp, is characterized by red papules, or spots, at the opening of the hair follicles. (Fig. 4.26) The patches spread and the hair becomes brittle and lifeless. It breaks off, leaving a stump, or falls from the enlarged open follicles.

Tinea favosa (fa-**VO**-sah), also *favus* (**FAY**-vus) or **honeycomb ringworm,** is characterized by dry, sulfur-yellow, cuplike crusts on the scalp, called *scutula* (**SKUT**-u-la), which have a peculiar odor. (Fig. 4.27) Scars from favus are bald patches that may be pink or white and shiny. It is *very contagious* and should be referred to a physician.

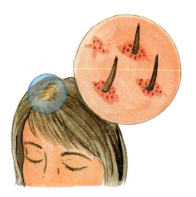

4.26—Tinea capitis.

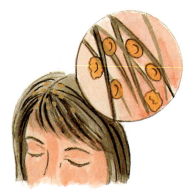

4.27—Favus.

ANIMAL PARASITIC INFECTIONS

Scabies "itch" is a highly contagious, animal parasitic skin disease, caused by the itch mite. Vesicles and pustules can form from the irritation of the parasites or from scratching the affected areas.

Pediculosis (pe-dik-yoo-**LOH**-sis) *capitis* is a contagious condition caused by the **head louse** (animal parasite) infesting the hair of the scalp. (Fig. 4.28) As the parasites feed on the scalp, itching occurs and the resultant scratching can cause an infection. The head louse is transmitted from one person to another by contact with infested hats, combs, brushes, or other personal articles. To kill head lice, advise the client to apply larkspur tincture, or other similar medication, to the entire head before retiring. The next morning, the client should shampoo with germicidal soap. Treatment should be repeated as necessary. Never treat a head lice condition in the salon or school.

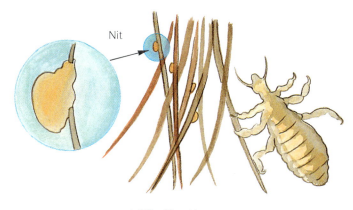

4.28—Head louse.

STAPHYLOCOCCI INFECTIONS

Furuncle (fu-**RUN**-kel), or boil, is an acute staphylococci infection of a hair follicle that produces constant pain. (Fig. 4.29) It is limited to a specific area and produces a pustule perforated by a hair.

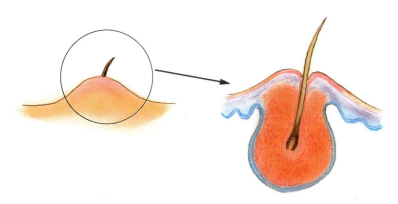

4.29—Furuncle (boil).

Carbuncle (**KAHR**-bun-kul) is the result of an acute staphylococci infection and is larger than a furuncle. Refer the client to a physician.

GENERAL HAIR AND SCALP TREATMENTS

The purpose of a general scalp treatment is to keep the scalp and hair in a clean and healthy condition. Regular scalp treatments also are beneficial in preventing baldness.

Procedure for Normal Hair and Scalp

1. Drape client.
2. Brush hair for about 5 minutes.
3. Apply scalp cream.
4. Apply infrared lamp for about 5 minutes. (Fig. 4.30)
5. Give scalp manipulations for 10 to 20 minutes.
6. Shampoo the hair.
7. Towel-dry the hair to remove excess moisture.
8. Apply suitable scalp lotion.
9. Set, dry, and style hair.
10. Clean up your workstation.

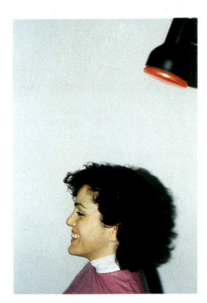

4.30—Applying heat with infrared lamp.

Dry Hair and Scalp Treatments

This treatment should be used when there is a deficiency of natural oil on the scalp and hair. Select scalp preparations containing moisturizing and emollient materials. Avoid the use of strong soaps, preparations containing a mineral oil or sulfonated oil base, greasy preparations, and lotions with a high alcohol content.

1. Drape client.
2. Brush client's hair for about 5 minutes.
3. Apply the scalp preparation for this condition.
4. Apply the scalp steamer for 7 to 10 minutes, or wrap the head in warm steam towels for 7 to 10 minutes. (Fig. 4.31)
5. Give a mild shampoo.
6. Towel dry the hair and scalp thoroughly.
7. Apply moisturizing scalp cream sparingly with a rotary, frictional motion.
8. Stimulate the scalp with direct high-frequency current, using the glass rake electrode, for about 5 minutes.
9. Set, dry, and style the hair.
10. Clean up your workstation.

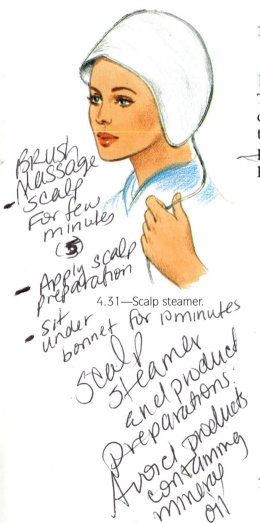

4.31—Scalp steamer.

Oily Hair and Scalp Treatments

Excessive oiliness is caused by the over-activity of the sebaceous (oil) glands. Manipulate the scalp and knead it to increase the blood circulation to the scalp. Any hardened sebum in the pores of the scalp will be removed with the correct degree of pressing and squeezing. To normalize the function of these glands, excess sebum should be flushed out with each treatment.

1. Drape client.
2. Brush client's hair for about 5 minutes.
3. Apply a medicated scalp lotion to the scalp only with a cotton pledget. (Fig. 4.32)
4. Apply infrared lamp for about 5 minutes.
5. Give scalp manipulations. (Optional: Faradic or sinusoidal current may be used.) (Figs. 4.33a, 4.33b)
6. Shampoo with a corrective shampoo for oily scalp.
7. Towel dry the hair.
8. Apply direct high-frequency current for 3 to 5 minutes.
9. Apply a scalp astringent.
10. Set, dry, and style the hair.
11. Clean up your workstation.

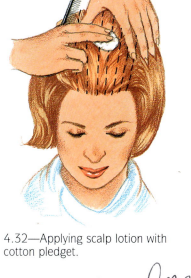

4.32—Applying scalp lotion with cotton pledget.

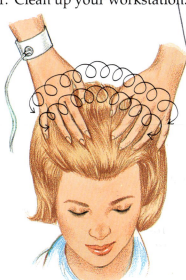

4.33a—Applying faradic current, cosmetologist manipulates the scalp.

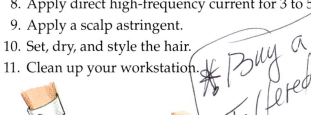

4.33b—While cosmetologist manipulates scalp, client holds the electrode.

CAUTION
Do not use high-frequency current on hair treated with tonics or lotions having alcohol content.

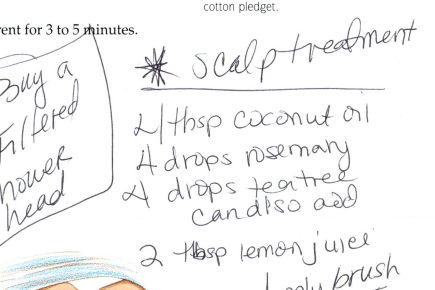

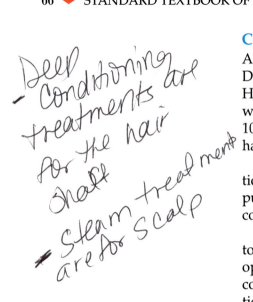
- Deep conditioning treatments are for the hair shaft
- Steam treatments are for scalp

Corrective Hair Treatment

A corrective hair treatment deals with the hair shaft, not the scalp. Dry and damaged hair can be greatly improved by conditioners. Hair treatments are especially beneficial and extremely important when given approximately a week or 10 days before, and a week or 10 days after, a permanent wave, tint, lightener, toner, or chemical hair straightening treatment.

Dry hair may be softened quickly with a conditioning preparation applied directly on the hair shaft. The product used for this purpose is usually an emulsion containing cholesterol and related compounds.

Some conditioners function more effectively when heat is applied to induce penetration into the cortex. The heat applied to the hair opens the cuticle's imbrications, and permits significantly more corrective agents to enter the hair shaft. This provides more conditioning benefits.

1. Drape client.
2. Brush the client's hair for about 5 minutes.
3. Apply a mild shampoo.
4. Towel dry the hair.
5. Apply a conditioner according to the manufacturer's directions.
6. Set, dry, and style hair.
7. Clean up your workstation. ✔

✔ **Completed—Learning Objective No. 12**

SCALP AND HAIR DISORDERS AND THEIR TREATMENTS

REVIEW QUESTIONS

PROPERTIES OF THE SCALP AND HAIR

1. What is the purpose of hair? page 44.
2. What is hair? page 45
3. What is hair composed of? page 45
4. What are the two principal parts of hair? page 45
5. What factors influence hair growth? page 49
6. What are the theories relating to the life and density of hair? page 49.
7. What determines the color of a person's hair? page 50
8. What is the basic requisite for a healthy scalp? page 52

DRAPING

5

LEARNING OBJECTIVES

AFTER COMPLETING THIS CHAPTER, YOU SHOULD BE ABLE TO:

1. List the methods of draping and preparing the client for cosmetology services.
2. Demonstrate draping for wet hair services.
3. Demonstrate draping for chemical services.
4. Demonstrate draping for dry hair services.

INTRODUCTION

The comfort and protection of the client must always be considered during cosmetology services. Protection of the skin and clothing assures clients that the cosmetologist is personally and professionally concerned about their comfort and safety.

Methods of draping depend on the service being performed. Several procedures are presented in this text, although those taught by your instructor are also acceptable. Consideration for the client is one of your most important responsibilities as a cosmetologist.

The following instructions are important before draping a client for any type of service:

1. Prepare materials and supplies for the service.
2. Sanitize hands.
3. Ask the client to remove all neck and hair jewelry and store it away.
4. Remove objects from the client's hair.
5. Turn the client's collar to the inside. (See Fig. 5.1)
6. Proceed with the appropriate draping method.

In the following procedures the purpose of the towel or neck strip is for sanitary reasons, to prevent contact of the cape with the client's skin.

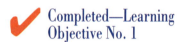

METHODS OF DRAPING AND PREPARING THE CLIENT FOR SERVICES

DRAPING FOR WET HAIR SERVICES

Shampooing, Scalp and Hair Care, and Haircutting

1. Place a towel lengthwise across the client's shoulders, crossing the ends beneath the chin.
2. Place the cape over the towel and fasten in the back so that the cape does not touch the client's skin.
3. Place another towel over the cape and secure in front.

For haircutting, the towel should be removed after shampooing and replaced with a neck strip. This allows the hair to fall naturally without obstruction.

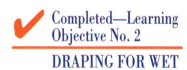

DRAPING FOR WET HAIR SERVICES

DRAPING FOR CHEMICAL SERVICES

Hair Color, Perms, and Relaxers

1. Slide towel down from back of client's head and place lengthwise across the client's shoulders. (See Fig. 5.2)

2. Cross the ends of the towel beneath the chin and place the cape over the towel. Fasten in the back and adjust the towel over the cape. (See Fig. 5.3)

3. Fold the towel over the top of the cape and secure in front. (See Fig. 5.4)

4. It is advisable to apply a protective cream around the hairline immediately prior to the application of chemicals to the hair. This prevents possible skin irritation.

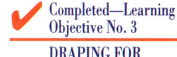
Completed—Learning Objective No. 3

DRAPING FOR CHEMICAL SERVICES

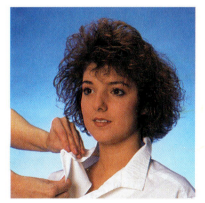
5.1—Turning collar in.

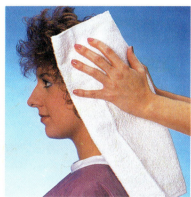
5.2—Sliding towel down around client's neck.

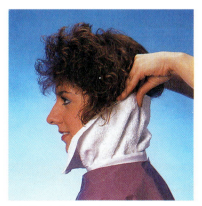
5.3—Adjusting towel over cape.

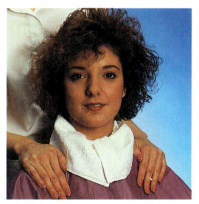
5.4—Folding towel over.

DRAPING FOR DRY HAIR SERVICES

Brushing or Thermal Design

1. Secure a neck strip around the client's neck. (See Fig. 5.5)
2. Place the cape over the neck strip and fasten so that the cape does not touch the client's skin. (See Fig. 5.6)
3. Fold the uncovered portion of the neck strip down over the cape. Make sure that no part of the cape touches the client's neck. (See Fig. 5.7)

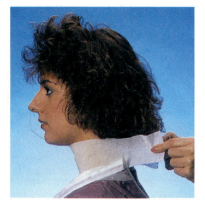
5.5—Placing neck strip.

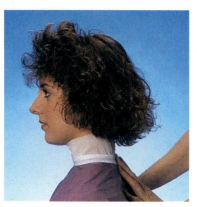
5.6—Placing cape over neck strip.

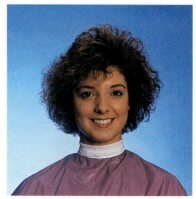
5.7—Folding neck strip down over cape.

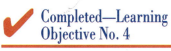

Completed—Learning Objective No. 4

DRAPING FOR DRY HAIR SERVICES

Comb-Out

1. Secure a neck strip around the client's neck.
2. Place the cape over the neck strip and fasten so that the cape does not touch the client's skin. (See Fig. 5.8) Capes especially designed for this service can be used.

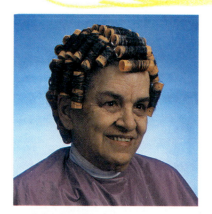
5.8—Draping for a comb-out.

Promo Power

THE IN-SALON PROMO

Promotions are great business. They can cause excitement among existing clients, while bringing in new ones.

Set the rules and regulations of any contests. Plan contests at least three months ahead of time so that you are able to do everything and have everything made. Decide on all of the features and benefits of the contest to the salon. List all the pros and cons, and plan for the worst-case scenario to make sure expenses could still be covered; then have a staff meeting to inform your people what you're planning and get their input. Without their consent and participation, you could have a mess on your hands. Excite them about the idea, and reward them with something that will be exciting to them. Staff prizes could be educational classes, bonuses, time off, or something that has meaning to an individual.

The planning stages of your promo are most important. All of the preparations must be thoroughly thought out and prioritized. It's important to know that everything is ready to go at least a couple of weeks ahead of time so people are aware of what is happening. At the actual time of the promo, follow up and keep your staff updated about what is happening on a daily or weekly basis.

—*From* The Salon Biz: Tips for Success *by Geri Mataya*

REVIEW QUESTIONS

DRAPING

1. What must a cosmetologist take into consideration when performing any service? *page 68*
2. What is draping?
3. Why is draping so important?
4. Why is a towel or neck strip used in draping? *page 68*
5. What are the four preliminary steps before draping a client? *page 68*
6. What are the differences when draping for wet hair services, dry hair services, and chemical services? *page 68-70*

SHAMPOOING, RINSING, AND CONDITIONING

6

LEARNING OBJECTIVES

AFTER COMPLETING THIS CHAPTER, YOU SHOULD BE ABLE TO:

1. List the reasons for good hygienic care of the hair and scalp.
2. Identify when, why, and how to brush hair.
3. Demonstrate the procedure for shampoo manipulations.
4. Understand the meaning of pH levels in shampoos.
5. Identify the various types of shampoos.
6. Identify the various types of rinses.

INTRODUCTION

Shampooing is the first step of a great many salon services, and a good shampoo sets the stage for a successful salon visit. In salons where the stylist gives the shampoo, the client may use this initial experience to evaluate the professional expertise of the stylist. Clients assume that the stylist who shampoos with a high level of professionalism will perform all additional services at that same level of competency and concern. In salons where there is a separate shampoo person, the client may use the experience to judge the professionalism of the salon. Therefore, the client who enjoys the shampoo service is more likely to request additional services and recommend the stylist and the salon to potential clients.

Shampooing is an important preliminary step for a variety of hair services and is given primarily to cleanse the hair and scalp. However, the psychological effects of a pleasurable and relaxing experience at the shampoo bowl will help to ensure that the client visits the salon on a regular basis.

To be effective, a shampoo must remove all dirt, oils, cosmetics, and skin debris without adversely affecting either the scalp or hair. It is important to analyze the condition of the client's hair and scalp and to check for disease or disorders. A client with an infectious disease should not be treated in the salon and should be referred to a physician.

Unless the scalp and hair are cleansed regularly, the accumulations of oil and perspiration, which mix with the natural scales and dirt, offer a breeding place for disease-producing bacteria. This can lead to scalp disorders.

Completed—Learning Objective No. 1

REASONS FOR GOOD HYGIENIC CARE OF HAIR AND SCALP

Hair should be shampooed as often as necessary, depending on how quickly the scalp and hair become soiled. As a general rule, oily hair should be shampooed more often than normal or dry hair.

WATER

Chemically, water is composed of hydrogen and oxygen (H_2O). Depending on the kinds and quantities of other minerals present, it can be classified as either hard or soft water. You will be able to make a more professional shampoo selection if you know whether the salon water is hard or soft.

Soft water is rain water or water that has been chemically softened. It contains small amounts of minerals and, therefore, allows shampoos to lather freely. For this reason, it may be preferred for shampooing.

Hard water contains certain minerals that lessen the ability of shampoo to lather. However, it can be softened by a chemical process.

SELECTING THE CORRECT SHAMPOO

Many types of shampoos are available. As a professional cosmetologist, you should learn the composition and action of a shampoo to determine whether or not it will serve your intended purpose. Read the label and accompanying literature carefully so that you can make an informed decision.

Select the shampoo according to the condition of the hair. Hair is not considered normal if it has been:

Lightened	Abused by the use of harsh shampoos
Toned or tinted	Damaged by improper care
Permanent waved	Damaged by exposure to the elements
Chemically relaxed	such as sun, cold, heat, wind

REQUIRED MATERIALS AND IMPLEMENTS

Prior to giving a shampoo, gather all necessary materials and implements. Don't forget that the client should be properly draped. The relaxing mood and the professional quality of the shampoo is destroyed if you dash off to get a forgotten item, leaving the client wet and dripping in the shampoo bowl. Required materials and implements are:

Towels	Hair rinse (optional)
Shampoo cape	Neck strip
Shampoo	Comb and hairbrush

BRUSHING

Hairbrushes made of natural bristles are recommended for hair brushing. Natural bristles have many tiny overlapping layers, or scales, which clean and add luster to the hair, while nylon bristles are shiny and smooth and recommended for hairstyling.

You should include a thorough hair brushing as a part of every shampoo and scalp treatment, with the following exceptions:

1. Do not brush before giving a chemical service.
2. Do not brush if the scalp is irritated.

Brushing stimulates the blood circulation to the scalp, helps remove dust, dirt, and hair spray buildup from the hair, and gives hair added sheen. (Fig. 6.1) Therefore, you should brush the hair whether the scalp and hair are in a dry or oily condition. Do not use the comb to loosen scales from the scalp.

To brush the hair, first part it through the center from front to nape. Then part a section about ½" (1.25 cm) off the center parting to the crown of the head. Holding this strand of hair in the left

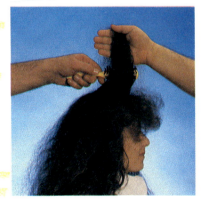

6.1—Brushing the hair.

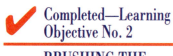

Completed—Learning Objective No. 2

BRUSHING THE HAIR

hand between the thumb and fingers, lay the brush (held in the right hand) with the bristles well down on the hair close to the scalp; rotate the brush by turning the wrist slightly, and sweep the bristles the full length of the hair shaft. Repeat three times. Then part the hair again ½" (1.25 cm) from the first parting and continue until the entire head has been brushed. ✔

SHAMPOO PROCEDURE

Preparation

1. Seat your client comfortably at your workstation.
2. Select and arrange the required materials.
3. Wash your hands.
4. Place a neck strip and shampoo cape around the client's neck. (Be sure that the client's collar lies smoothly under the garment before the neck strip is adjusted or turn collar to inside of garment.)
5. Remove all hairpins and combs from the hair.
6. Ask client to remove earrings and glasses and to put them in a safe place.
7. Examine the condition of the client's hair and scalp.
8. Brush the hair thoroughly.
9. Re-drape with shampoo cape and towel.
10. Seat the client comfortably at the shampoo sink.
11. Adjust the shampoo cape over the back of the shampoo chair. (Fig. 6.2)
12. Adjust the volume and temperature of the water spray.

Consider the client's preference in adjusting the water temperature. Turn on the cold water first and gradually add warm water until you obtain a comfortably warm temperature. The temperature of the water must be constantly monitored by keeping one finger over the edge of the spray nozzle and in contact with the water.

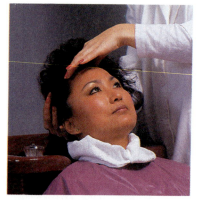

6.2—Support client's head with your right hand and place the cape over the back of the chair.

Procedure

1. **Saturate, wet hair thoroughly,** with warm water spray. Lift the hair and work it with your free hand to saturate the scalp. Shift your hand to protect the client's face, ears, and neck from the spray when working around the hairline. (Figs. 6.3–6.5)
2. **Apply small quantities of shampoo to the hair,** beginning at the hairline and working back. Work into a lather using the pads or cushions of the fingers.

CHAPTER 6   SHAMPOOING, RINSING, AND CONDITIONING   ◆   77

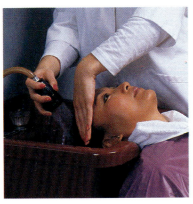
6.3—Protecting the face.

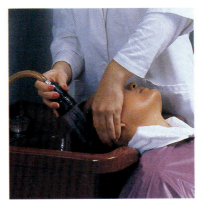
6.4—Protecting the ears.

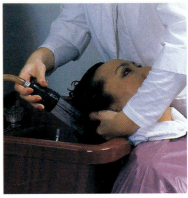
6.5—Protecting the neck.

Reminders

In massaging the scalp, do not use firm pressure if:

- You will be giving the client a chemical service after the shampoo.
- The client's scalp is tender or sensitive.
- The client requests less pressure.

3. ***Manipulate scalp.***

   a) Begin at the front hairline and work in a back-and-forth movement until the top of the head is reached. (See Fig. 6.6)

   b) Continue in this manner to the back of the head, shifting your fingers back 1" (2.5 cm) at a time.

   c) Lift the client's head, with your left hand controlling the movement of the head. With your right hand, start at the top of the right ear and, using the same movement, work to the back of the head. (See Fig. 6.7)

   d) Drop your fingers down 1" (2.5 cm) and repeat the process until the right side of the head is covered.

   e) Beginning at the left ear, repeat steps c and d.

   f) Allow the client's head to relax and work around the hairline with your thumbs in a rotary movement.

   g) Repeat these movements until the scalp has been thoroughly massaged.

   h) Remove excess shampoo and lather by squeezing the hair.

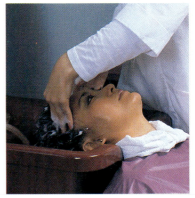
6.6—Manipulating scalp.

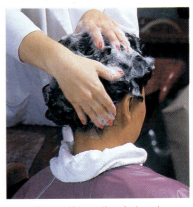
6.7—Lifting client's head.

4. *Rinse hair thoroughly* with a strong spray.
    a) Lift the hair at the crown and back with the fingers of your left hand to permit the spray to rinse the hair thoroughly.
    b) Cup your left hand along the napeline and pat the hair, forcing the spray of water against the base scalp area.
5. *If required, apply shampoo again.*
    a) Repeat the procedure using steps 2, 3, and 4 as outlined. You will need less shampoo because partially clean hair lathers more easily.
6. *Partially towel dry.*
    a) Remove excess moisture from the hair at the shampoo bowl.
    b) Wipe excess moisture from around the client's face and ears with the ends of the towel.
    c) Lift the towel over the back of the client's head and drape the head with the towel.
    d) Place your hands on top of the towel and massage until the hair is partially dry. (Fig. 6.8)

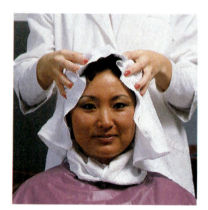

6.8—Towel drying the hair.

Completion

1. Comb the hair, beginning with the ends at the nape of the client's neck.
2. Change the drape if necessary.
3. Style the hair as desired.

Cleanup

1. Discard used materials, and place unused supplies in their proper place.
2. Place used towels in the towel hamper.
3. Remove hair from combs and brushes; wash with hot, soapy water; rinse; and place in wet disinfectant for the required time.
4. Sanitize the shampoo bowl.
5. Cleanse your hands. ✔

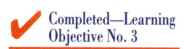

Completed—Learning Objective No. 3

PROCEDURE FOR SHAMPOO MANIPULATIONS

SHAMPOOING CHEMICALLY TREATED HAIR

Chemically treated hair tends to be drier and more fragile than non-chemically treated hair. Therefore, a mild shampoo formulated for chemically treated hair is recommended. Chemically treated hair also tends to tangle. To remove tangles, comb gently from the nape of the head and work to the frontal area. Do not force the comb through the hair. Use a conditioner if necessary.

TYPES OF SHAMPOOS

Shampoo accounts for the highest dollar expenditure in hair care products. Consumer studies show the current growth pattern in the shampoo market to be in the direction of the professional salon. You will have to be more knowledgeable and sophisticated about the products used, more proficient in using them, and capable of selling these products to your clients.

Thousands of good shampoos exist, one for every conceivable type of hair or scalp condition a client could have: dry, oily, fine, coarse, limp, lightened, permed, relaxed, or chemically untreated. There are shampoos that add highlights and others that remove them. There are shampoos that deposit a coating on the hair, and there are shampoos which strip coating off the hair.

The ingredients list is the key to determining which shampoo will leave a client's hair lustrous and manageable, treat a scalp or hair condition, or prepare hair for chemical treatment. Most shampoos have many common ingredients, and it is your responsibility as a professional cosmetologist to understand the chemical composition in order to select the best shampoo for each particular service and client.

General descriptions of different types of shampoos are listed below. The section entitled "Chemistry of Shampoos" in the chapter on chemistry has detailed information about the chemical ingredients that make up the different types of shampoos.

Explaining pH

Before discussing acid-balanced shampoos, you should know something about pH (potential hydrogen) levels in shampoo. This will help you to select the proper shampoo for your client. The amount of hydrogen in a solution is measured on a pH scale that has a range from 0 to 14. The amount of hydrogen in a solution determines whether it is more alkaline or more acid. A shampoo that is more acid can have a pH rating from 0 to 6.9; a shampoo that is more alkaline can have a pH rating from 7 to 14. The higher the pH rating (more alkaline), the stronger and harsher the shampoo is to the hair. A high pH shampoo can leave the hair dry and brittle. (Also see pH scale in the chapter on chemistry.)

Acid-balanced Shampoos

An acid-balanced shampoo is one that falls within the 4.5 to 6.6 range, an acceptable pH range. Any shampoo can become acid balanced by the addition of citric, lactic, or phosphoric acid.

Proponents of acid-balanced shampoo state that an acid pH of 4.5 to 5.5 is essential to prevent excessive dryness and hair damage during the cleansing process, while the Consumer's Union's chemists consider the difference between a pH of 5 and a pH of 8 too small to affect the hair and scalp in the limited time of an average application.

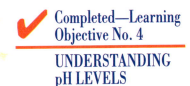

Completed—Learning Objective No. 4

UNDERSTANDING pH LEVELS

Question & Answer

CLEANSING

Q: *During a routine shampoo service some of the shampoo accidentally went into the eye of a client. She complained of burning, and the eye turned extremely red. What should I do in such a case?*

A: Strong synthetics in some shampoos—those containing cationics as germicides and nonionics as cleansing agents—are indeed capable of causing severe eye irritation and even permanent eye injury. Most manufacturers do not make this type of shampoo, however. Any shampoo, unless it is specifically made for use on babies and children, will cause temporary discomfort if it comes in direct contact with the eye. However, there are no documented cases of severe or lasting injury from other shampoos.

First and foremost, know your products. Purchase high-quality shampoo products that have proven effective and safe over a sufficient period of time.

Then, care in executing the cleansing service is necessary. No client wants suds and water in her face, even if it is not harmful. Scalp manipulations for shampooing purposes should be methodical but always confined to the hair portion of the head.

If shampoo accidentally gets into the client's eye, put the client in an upright position and immediately rinse the eye with clear, cold water. Allow the client to rinse her own eye to avoid rubbing beyond her personal tolerance. Blot the area dry. If the redness persists, ask the client if she would like to see her doctor; if so the salon will gladly pay for the office visit and initial treatment. Notify your insurance company at once so they can follow up if there's a problem. The law holds the manufacturer of synthetic detergent shampoo or other cosmetics solely responsible for users' safety. However, you have a co-responsibility to use it in a safe manner—only for its intended purpose.

—*From* Milady's Salon Solutions *by Louise Cotter*

Conditioning Shampoos

Virtually every shampoo available on the professional market contains one or more conditioning agents designed to make the hair smooth and shiny, to avoid damage to chemically treated hair, and to improve the manageability of the hair. Protein, dimethicone, biotin, hydantoin, oleyl alcohol, and cocoamphocarboxyglycinate are just a few examples of conditioning agents that are used to assist shampoos in meeting current grooming needs.

Medicated Shampoos

Medicated shampoos contain special chemicals or drugs that are very effective in reducing excessive dandruff or other scalp conditions. These are prescribed by a physician. They generally are quite strong and will affect the color of tinted or lightened hair.

Powder Dry Shampoos

A dry shampoo is usually given when the client's health does not permit a wet shampoo. Only a few of these products are available on the market today. Follow the manufacturer's recommended directions when giving a dry shampoo. Do not give a dry shampoo before performing a chemical service. (Fig. 6.9)

Color or Highlighting Shampoos

(See chapters on hair coloring and chemistry.)

Shampoos for Hairpieces and Wigs

Prepared wig cleaning solutions are now available. (See chapter on the artistry of artificial hair.) ✓

HAIR RINSES

A hair rinse consists of a mixture of water with a mild acid, coloring agent, or ingredients designed to serve a particular purpose. (Fig. 6.10)

Acid Rinses

Acid rinses are used to restore the pH balance to the hair and to remove soap scum. The fatty acids found in soap combine with the minerals in water to form a soap scum that cannot be completely removed from the hair with plain water. Therefore, the hair tends to become coated, dull, and difficult to comb. Because soap is not currently used in the manufacture of professional shampoos, you will not find acid rinses in many salons.

The types of acids used in prepared acid hair rinses are:

Citric acid from the juice of a lime, orange, or lemon.

Tartaric acid, which is obtained from residues in wine making.

Acetic acid, which is present in vinegar.

Lactic acid, which is lactose or sugar of milk.

Conditioners and Cream Rinses

A conditioner or cream rinse is a commercial product with a creamy appearance that is used after shampooing. It is intended to soften hair, add luster, and make tangled hair easier to comb. Conditioners and cream rinses coat the hair shaft to make it slick and smooth. This temporary coating allows the comb to glide easily through the hair and often gives the false impression that the hair has been restored to its original healthy condition.

Used occasionally, conditioners and cream rinses are useful to remove tangles. However, habitual use can lead to future hair care problems. The coating ingredients can build up on the hair, making it prematurely heavy and oily. This can lead the client to shampoo more frequently, causing further damage to the hair. An endless

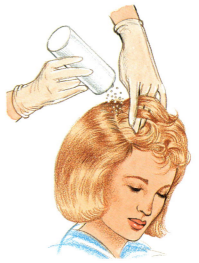

6.9—Applying powder dry shampoo.

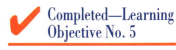

✓ Completed—Learning Objective No. 5

TYPES OF SHAMPOOS

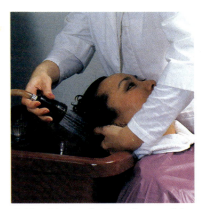

6.10—Rinsing the hair after applying a hair rinse.

cycle is created because conditioners and cream rinses give the illusion of curing a problem that they are actually compounding. Professional conditioning treatments are an effective solution to the problem.

Acid-balanced Rinses

Acid-balanced rinses are commercially formulated to prevent the fading of color after a tint or toner application and to give shine. This rinse is acid balanced to close the cuticle and trap within it the color molecules. This helps to prevent fading. Citric acid is probably the most commonly used ingredient in an after-rinse, but most also contain a mild moisturizer to leave the hair soft, pliable, and easy to comb.

Medicated Rinses

Medicated rinses are formulated to control minor dandruff conditions. Follow the manufacturer's instructions.

Color Rinses

Color rinses highlight or add temporary color to the hair. These rinses remain on the hair until the next shampoo. (For additional information, see the chapter on hair coloring.)

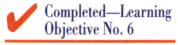

Completed—Learning Objective No. 6

TYPES OF RINSES

REVIEW QUESTIONS

SHAMPOOING, RINSING, AND CONDITIONING

1. Why is a professional shampoo important? page 74
2. What is the purpose of a shampoo? 74
3. Why and how often should the hair be shampooed? 74
4. How do you determine the proper shampoo to use? 75
5. Name two types of water. 74
6. Why is brushing important prior to shampooing? 75
7. When is it not appropriate to brush before shampooing? 75
8. What does pH mean? 79
9. How is pH measured? 79
10. Why is pH in shampoo important? 79
11. What is a hair rinse? 81
12. What is the function of an acid rinse? 81
13. What type of rinse is intended to soften the hair, add luster, and remove tangles? 81
14. What type of rinse prevents fading of color after a tint or toner application? 82
15. How does an acid-balanced rinse prevent fading? 82
16. What is a medicated rinse? 82
17. What is the purpose of a color rinse? 82

HAIRCUTTING

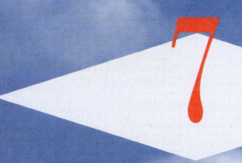

LEARNING OBJECTIVES

AFTER COMPLETING THIS CHAPTER, YOU SHOULD BE ABLE TO:

1. Describe why professional haircutting is a foundation for hairstyling and other services performed in the salon.

2. Demonstrate proper hair sectioning and its relationship to professional haircutting.

3. Explain the correct use of basic haircutting implements.

4. List the various techniques used in hair thinning.

5. List the basic techniques for cutting with scissors or with a razor.

INTRODUCTION

As a cosmetology student, you will learn to master the art and techniques of *haircutting*. Your haircutting skills will increase your professional qualifications in the salon. Thorough instruction is required in the proper way to cut and shape the hair, using a regular scissors, thinning shears, or a razor. Instruction must be followed by continual practice under the guidance of an instructor. A good haircut serves as a foundation for attractive hairstyles and for other services performed in the salon. A cosmetology education is not complete until you have acquired the artistic skill and judgment necessary for successful haircutting.

Hairstyles should accentuate the client's good points while minimizing his or her poor features. In selecting a suitable hairstyle, take into consideration the client's head shape, facial contour, neckline, and hair texture. However, you should also be guided by the client's wishes, personality, and lifestyle.

IMPLEMENTS USED IN HAIRCUTTING

The quality and selection of implements is important in order to accomplish a good haircut. To do your best work, the cosmetology student should buy and use only superior implements from a reliable manufacturer. However, improper use will quickly destroy the efficiency of any implement, no matter how perfectly it might be made at the factory.

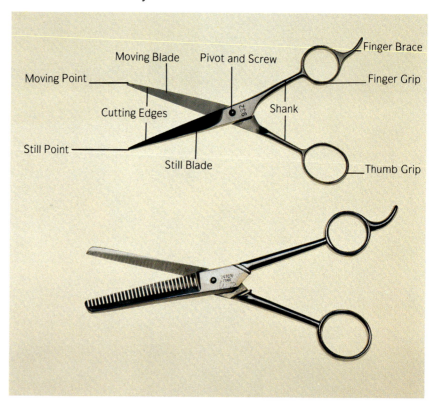

7.1—Haircutting scissors (top); thinning shears, one blade notched (bottom).

The following are the implements used in haircutting (Figs. 7.1, 7.2):

Regular haircutting scissors
Thinning shears (single- or double-notched blades)

Razors with safety guards
Hair clippers (See Fig. 7.33)
Combs and clippies (See Fig. 9.1 for illustrations of clippies) ✔

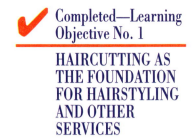

✔ **Completed—Learning Objective No. 1**

HAIRCUTTING AS THE FOUNDATION FOR HAIRSTYLING AND OTHER SERVICES

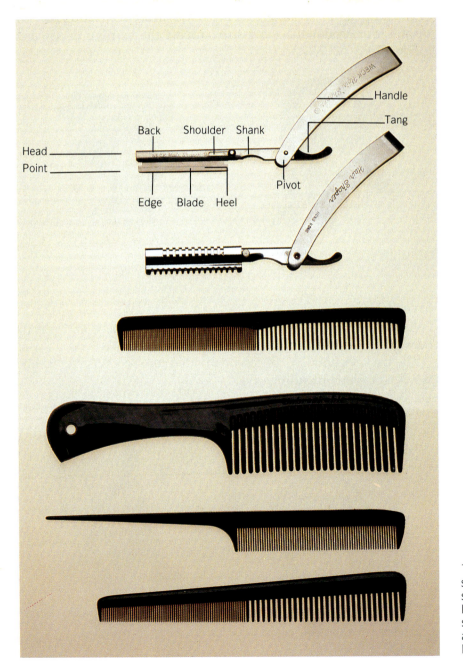

7.2—From top to bottom: straight razor; straight razor with safety guards; all-purpose comb; large-tooth comb; tail comb; hair shaping comb. Note: Tail combs are not allowed in all states for haircutting.

SECTIONING FOR HAIRCUTTING

By following a practical step-by-step procedure, you will soon learn how to give a professional haircut. The first step is to section the hair properly. The following illustrations cover the practical and accepted methods for dividing the hair into either four or five sections. In any case, follow your instructor's methods for dry or wet haircutting.

Four-Section Parting

Part hair down the center from the forehead to the *nape* (the back of the neck) and also across the top of the head from ear to ear. Pin up the four sections, leaving hair around the hairline to use as a guide. (Figs. 7.3, 7.4)

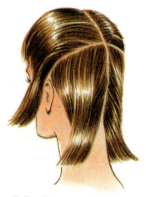
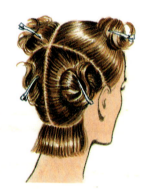

7.3—Four-section parting.   7.4—Four-section with guideline.

Five-Section Parting

Five-section parting with subparting panels: section and pin up hair in the order shown in the illustrations.

The back section (No. 5) can be divided into sections No. 5a and No. 5b for easier handling. (Figs. 7.5–7.7)

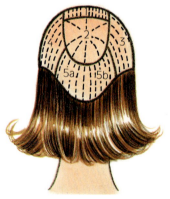
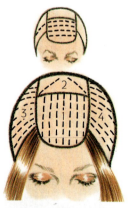
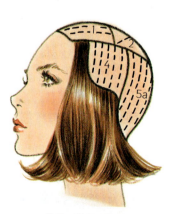

7.5—Back view.   7.6—Top section No. 1 may be subparted either in a horizontal or vertical direction.   7.7—Side view.

Alternative Five-Section Method

Another way to divide the hair into five sections is to part the hair across the *crown* (the top part of the head) from ear to ear, then subdivide the hair in the same order as shown in the illustration. (Fig. 7.8)

HOLDING HAIR SHAPING IMPLEMENTS

Scissors (Shears)

Haircutting scissors are handled correctly by inserting the third (ring) finger into the ring of the still blade and placing the little finger on the finger brace. The thumb is inserted into the ring of the movable blade. The tip of the index finger is braced near the pivot of the scissors in order to have better control. (Fig. 7.9)

Thinning Shears

Excess bulk is easily removed from the hair with a thinning shear. As can be seen in Fig. 7.1, thinning shears are quite similar to haircutting scissors, except that they have one or both blades *notched* or *serrated*. The single-notched edge cuts more hair. Which one is used depends on the preference of the cosmetologist. The notches provide a way to thin the hair in a uniform manner. Both thinning shears and cutting scissors are held in the same way. (Figs. 7.10, 7.11)

Holding Comb and Scissors

During the haircutting process, you will be holding both comb and scissors. Practice by closing the blades of the scissors, removing the thumb from the ring, and resting the scissors in the palm. Hold the scissors securely with the ring finger. The comb is held between the thumb and fingers. (Fig. 7.12)

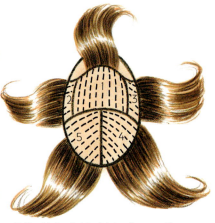

7.8—Hair divided into five sections with center back parting.

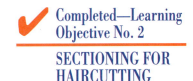

Completed—Learning Objective No. 2

SECTIONING FOR HAIRCUTTING

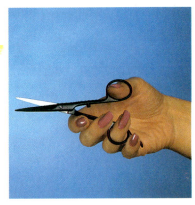

7.9—Holding scissors (shears).

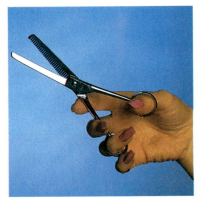

7.10—Holding thinning shears with one blade notched.

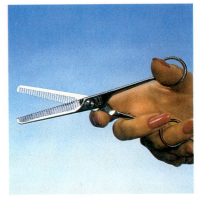

7.11—Holding thinning shears with both blades notched.

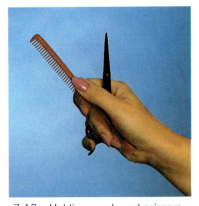

7.12—Holding comb and scissors.

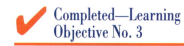

Completed—Learning Objective No. 3

USE OF BASIC HAIRCUTTING IMPLEMENTS

◆**NOTE:** When combing the hair, hold the comb and scissors in the right hand, as shown. When shaping (cutting) the hair, hold the comb in the left hand. To save time, do not put down the comb or scissors during shaping. ✔

HAIR THINNING

The purpose of *thinning* or *texturizing* hair is to remove excess bulk without shortening its length. For best results, use the following suggestions:

1. When using a razor for thinning or shaping, first dampen the hair.
2. When using thinning shears or regular scissors, the hair may be either dry or damp.

Hair texture determines the point where thinning should start on the hair strand. As a rule, fine hair may be thinned closer to the scalp than coarse hair. Fine hair is softer and more pliable, and when cut very short will lie flatter on the head. On the other hand, if coarse hair is thinned too close to the scalp, the short, stubby ends will protrude through the top layer.

The amount of hair you thin depends on the particular hairstyle. As a guide, start thinning different textures of hair as follows:

1. *Fine hair:* ½" to 1" (1.25 to 2.5 cm) from the scalp
2. *Medium hair:* 1" to 1½" (2.5 to 3.75 cm) from the scalp
3. *Coarse hair:* 1½" to 2" (3.75 to 5 cm) from the scalp

Hair Thinning Areas

There are several areas where it is *not* advisable to thin the hair (Fig. 7.13):

1. At the nape of the neck (ear to ear).
2. At the side of the head, above ears.
3. Around the facial hairline. Usually hair is not heavy at the hairline.
4. In the hair part. The cut ends will be seen in the finished hairstyle.

◆**NOTE:** Never thin the hair near the ends of a strand; to do so will render the hair shapeless.

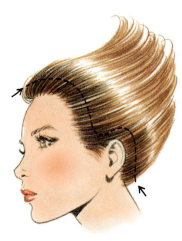

7.13—Dotted line shows hair that does not require thinning.

CHAPTER 7   HAIRCUTTING   ◆   89

> ### CAUTION
> During the thinning process, remember that you can always go back and remove more hair if necessary. However, once the hair has been cut, it is impossible to replace and you might have difficulty in achieving the desired hairstyle.

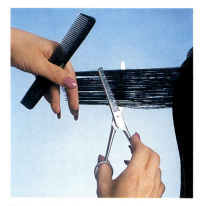

7.14—Thinning with thinning shears.

Thinning with Thinning Shears

When using the thinning shears, grip the hair firmly and evenly by overlapping the middle finger slightly over the index finger.

Procedure

1. Pick up a section of hair from ½" to 1" (1.25 to 2.5 cm) wide by 2" to 3" (5 to 7.5 cm) long, depending on the hair's texture.
2. Hold the section straight out from the scalp between the middle and index fingers.
3. Place thinning shears 1" to 2" (2.5 to 5 cm) from the scalp.
4. Cut the section by partly closing the thinning shears three-quarters through the strand. (Fig. 7.14)
5. Move out another 1½" (3.75 cm) and cut again.
6. Repeat if necessary.

◆ **NOTE:** It is advisable to avoid thinning the top part of the section.

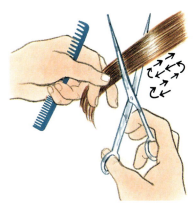

7.15—Thinning with haircutting scissors (shears).

Thinning with Haircutting Scissors (Shears)

When using regular haircutting scissors to thin the hair, pick up smaller sections of hair than when using the thinning shears. This process of thinning with scissors is known as *slithering* or *effilating*, and requires a different technique. (Fig. 7.15)

Procedure

1. Hold a section of hair straight out between the middle and index fingers.
2. Place the hair in the scissors so that only the underneath hair will be cut.
3. Slide the scissors about 1" to 1½" (2.5 to 3.75 cm) down the section, closing them slightly each time the scissors are moved toward the scalp.
4. Repeat this procedure twice on each section.

Alternate method: Hold the hair with the thumb and index finger. (Fig. 7.16)

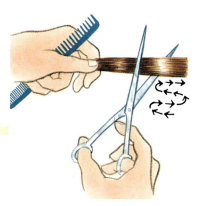

7.16—Holding the hair with thumb and index finger.

90 ◆ STANDARD TEXTBOOK OF COSMETOLOGY

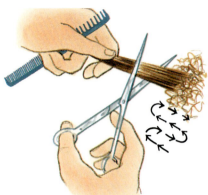

7.17—Slithering the hair after back-combing.

✔ **Completed—Learning Objective No. 4**

HAIR THINNING

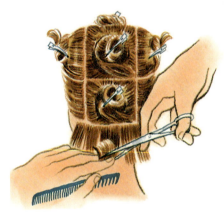

7.18—Blunt cutting strand at center nape to desired length.

Back-combing method: The short hair may be back-combed and then slithered. (Fig. 7.17)

HAIRCUTTING WITH SCISSORS

Scissor shaping can be done either on dry or wet hair.

Dry shaping. If hair is shaped while dry, it is recommended that you first shampoo and completely dry the hair prior to shaping.

Wet shaping. The hair can be shaped immediately after it has been shampooed.

Preparation

1. Seat the client; adjust the neck strip and plastic cape.
2. Analyze the head shape, facial features, and hair texture.
3. Decide on a suitable haircut with the client.
4. Comb and brush the hair free of tangles.

Procedure

1. Divide the hair into five sections.
2. Determine the length of the *nape guideline hair,* the section that will serve as a length guide while you cut the hair.
3. **Blunt cut** (cutting hair straight without slithering) the guideline strand of nape hair. (See Fig. 7.18)
   a) Blunt cut the strand on the left side, using the strand closest to the earlobe and using the earlobe as a guide. (See Fig. 7.19)
   b) Blunt cut the strand on the right side to match the left side.
   c) Blunt cut from back center to left front. (See Fig. 7.20)
   d) Blunt cut from back center to right front for completed guideline. (See Fig. 7.21)

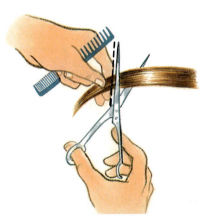

7.19—Blunt cutting.

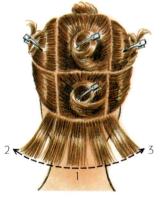

7.20—Following up by cutting all remaining guideline hair.

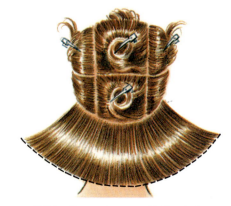

7.21—Properly cut guideline hair.

CHAPTER 7 HAIRCUTTING ◆ 91

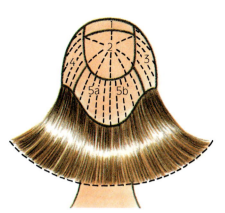

7.22—Divide section No. 5 into two equal parts.

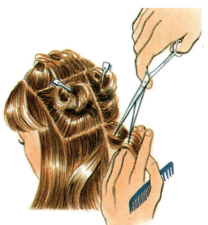

7.23—Blunt cutting section No. 5b.

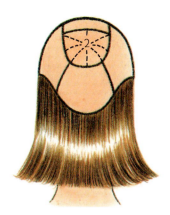

7.24—Crown section.

4. Let down section No. 5 and divide into two equal parts (No. 5a and No. 5b). Match length with guideline hair. (See Fig. 7.22) Either the left side or the right side may be done first. Hold hair panels out from the head while blunt cutting. (See Fig. 7.23) Continue cutting sections No. 3 and No. 4 in the same manner.

Crown Section

Crown section No. 2. Hold the pie-shaped strands out from the head; match length by picking up strands from the section already cut. Continue around the head, matching the length with sides and back hair. (See Figs. 7.24, 7.25)

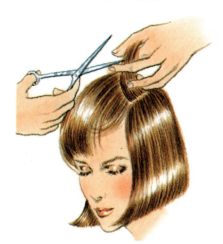

7.25—Shaping crown section.

Top Front Section

Divide section No. 1 into two parts. Pick up hair in the middle section using a few strands of previously cut hair from the crown as a guide. Maintain the hand movement in a 45° (.785 rad) arc. Proceed to cut both parts of section No. 1 in the prescribed manner. (See Figs. 7.26, 7.27)

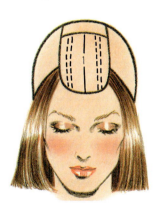

7.26—Top view section No. 1 with vertical partings.

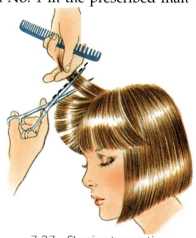

7.27—Shaping top section.

If bangs are to be cut, work directly in front of the client for even cutting. Test hair for bounce (elasticity), then determine the desired length. If the bangs are to be short, use the bridge of the nose as a guide. If the style is to be long, shape strands to blend into the length of the sides. (See Figs. 7.28–7.30)

Reducing bulk. To complete cutting the hair, remove excess bulk by thinning with a razor, thinning shears, or scissors. It is recommended that all hair be checked for proper length.

Question & Answer

PROBLEMS IN SHINGLING

Q *How can I give a shingled neckline on a client whose hair on the nape is sparse and does not grow low on the neck?*

A The only answer is to make the hair at the nape "fitted" in relation to other lengths in the hairstyle. Establish an adaptable hanging length at the nape, then use vertical partings so you can control the degree of graduation from the nape to the length you will use throughout. Instead of positioning your fingers so the hair will be "zero" at the hanging length, move the holding fingers about ½ inch away from the head and cut the hair from ½ to 2 inches at the occipital bone. When the haircut is finished you can use texture shears to remove excess bulk above the hanging guide. This method gives the illusion of a fitted back even when the hair doesn't start its growth at the established guide.

Q *How can I avoid getting visible steps when cutting hair very short in the back?*

A Because the scalp is flexible, it stretches when the head is bent forward and relaxes when the head is held upright; this can cause steps to appear when the client raises his or her head.

Cut the client's hair with the head in an upright position. Position your body lower than the client's head so your hands and shears are parallel with the floor. It is good to have at hand a low cutting stool for this purpose. Then, if you do not know the scissors-over-comb technique for shingling or cutting hair close, by all means learn quickly. The best teachers of the S.O.C. method are barbers or stylists working in an "all-male" salon.

—*From* Milady's Salon Solutions *by Louise Cotter*

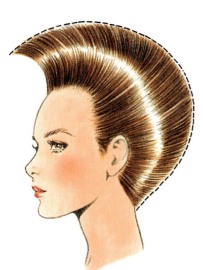
7.28—Correct uniform shaping.

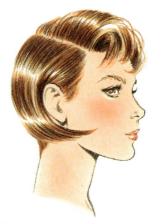
7.29—Completed shaping with bang effect and/or off-face style.

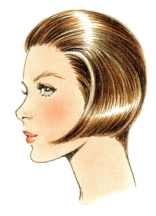
7.30—Hair shaping for straight back style.

Completion

Remove the neck strip and plastic cape. Thoroughly clean all hair clippings from the cape, client's clothing, and the work area. You may then proceed with the next professional service desired by the client.

SHINGLING

Shingling is cutting the hair close to the nape and gradually longer toward the crown, without showing a definite line.

Regardless of the current hair fashions, there will always be clients who prefer to have their hair cut short. To satisfy these clients, you must know how to shingle the hair. The accompanying illustrations show how to accomplish shingling with the use of shears and comb. (See Figs. 7.31, 7.32)

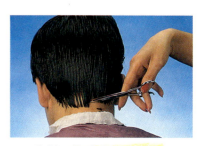
7.31—Outlining neckline.

Procedure

Shingling should be done at eye level. Start by outlining neckline. Hold the hair in the comb and cut upward in a graduated effect. When you reach the top of the section being shingled, turn the comb downward and comb the hair. Proceed, section by section, until the entire back of the head is shingled in a smooth, uniform manner.

◆ NOTE: In shingling, the blades of the scissors are held parallel with the comb; only the top blade moves and does the cutting.

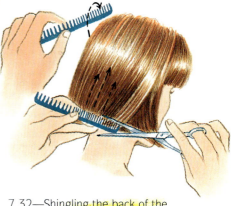
7.32—Shingling the back of the head.

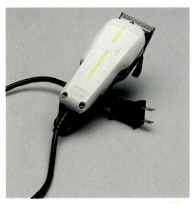

7.33—Electric haircutting clippers.

USE OF CLIPPERS ON THE NECKLINE

There is a mistaken notion that using clippers to "clean" the neckline makes the hair grow in thicker on the neck. This is not true, because the amount of human hair can only be as great as the number of follicles in the area. Use of clippers or any other implement does not increase the number of follicles. (Figs. 7.33, 7.34)

USING THE RAZOR

The successful cosmetologist must be versatile in handling all haircutting implements efficiently, including the straight razor.

How to Hold the Razor

Finger wrap hold. Place the thumb in the groove part of the **shank** and fold the fingers over the handle of the razor. The **guard** faces the cosmetologist while working. (See Fig. 7.35)

Three-finger hold. Place three fingers over the shank, the thumb in the groove of the shank, and the little finger in the hollow part of the tang. (See Fig. 7.36)

◆ **NOTE:** When combing the hair, hold the razor and comb in the right hand. (See Fig. 7.37) When cutting the hair with a razor, hold the comb in the left hand. Do not put down the comb or razor.

When using the razor, keep the hair damp to avoid pulling the hair and to prevent dulling the razor.

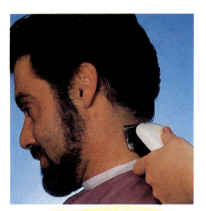

7.34—Cleaning the neck with clippers.

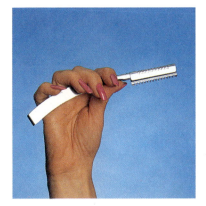

7.35—Finger wrap hold.

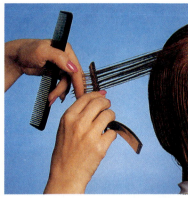

7.36—Blunt razor cutting using three-finger hold.

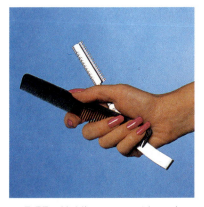

7.37—Holding razor and comb.

CHAPTER 7   HAIRCUTTING   ◆   95

Changing Blades

Removing an old blade. Remove the guard. With the left hand, hold the shaper firmly above the joint. Catch the blade in the teeth of the upper part of the guard and push out the blade. (See Fig. 7.38)

Inserting a new blade. Slide the blade into the groove, pushing the end carefully with your fingers. Place the tooth end of the guard into the blade notch and slide the blade in until it clicks into position. Slide the guard over the blade, making sure the free or open end is over the cutting edge of the blade.

Thinning with a Razor

Hold a strand of wet hair straight out between the middle and index fingers. Place the razor flat, not erect, about ½″ (1.25 cm) from the scalp (depending on the hair texture), and use short, steady strokes toward the hair ends. (See Figs. 7.39–7.41)

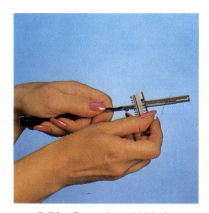
7.38—Removing old blade.

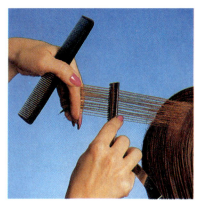
7.39—Thinning with razor.

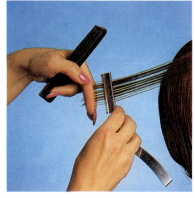
7.40—Tapering hair ends with razor.

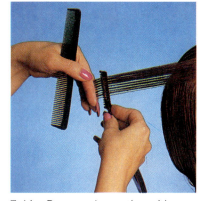
7.41—Razor under-cutting with upward stroke.

Haircutting with a Razor

Preparation

1. Seat the client; adjust the neck strip and plastic cape.
2. Analyze the head shape, facial features, and hair texture.
3. Decide on a suitable haircut with the client.
4. Comb and brush the hair free of tangles.
5. Shampoo and cut the hair while it is wet.

Procedure

1. Divide the hair into five sections.
2. Determine the length of the nape guideline hair.
3. Blunt cut a guideline strand of nape hair. (See Fig. 7.42)
   a) Blunt cut a strand on the left side; use the earlobe as a guide.
   b) Blunt cut a strand on the right side to match the left side.
   c) Use guideline hair to cut from the back center to the left front and back center to the right front. (See Fig. 7.43)
   d) Complete guideline. (See Fig. 7.44)

Cutting back sections No. 5a and No. 5b. Divide section No. 5 into two parts (sections No. 5a and No. 5b). From the center of section No. 5a, pick horizontal strands. Pick up a guideline strand for length. When guideline hair falls away, cut the hair, moving hands out and upward into a 45° (.785 rad) arc. (See Fig. 7.45)

Cutting section No. 4. Proceed to cut to the left into section No. 4 in the same manner.

Cutting section No. 3. Return to section No. 5b and cut this section, moving to the right into section No. 3, always lifting hands in an upward 45° (.785 rad) arc as the hair is cut. Measure carefully with guideline hair.

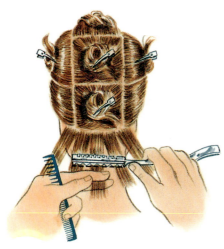

7.42—Blunt cutting a strand at center nape for desired hair length.

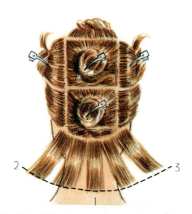

7.43—Following up by cutting all remaining guideline hair.

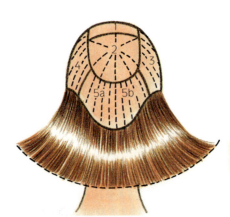

7.44—Completed guideline.

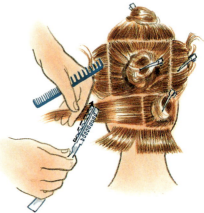

7.45—Shaping section No. 5a.

CHAPTER 7　HAIRCUTTING　◆　97

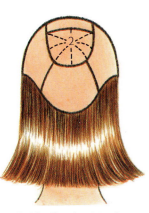

7.46—Section No. 2.

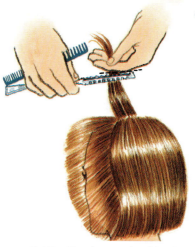

7.47—Shaping section No. 2.

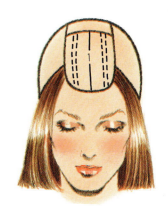

7.48—Section No. 1 shown with vertical parting.

Cutting section No. 2. Next, proceed to cut section No. 2 (crown), using the previously cut hair as a guide. (See Figs. 7.46, 7.47)

Cutting section 1. Divide section No. 1 into two parts. Pick up hair in the middle of the section using a few strands of previously cut hair from the crown as a guide. Maintain the hand movement in a 45° (.785 rad) arc. Proceed to cut both parts of section No. 1 in the prescribed manner. (See Figs. 7.48, 7.49)

Bangs. To cut bangs evenly, work directly in front of the client. Test hair for bounce (elasticity), then determine the desired length. If the bangs are to be short, use the bridge of the nose as a guide. If the style is to be long, shape strands to blend into the length of the sides.

Reducing bulk. To complete cutting the hair, remove excess bulk by thinning with a razor, thinning shears, or scissors. Be sure to check hair for proper length. (See Figs. 7.50, 7.51)

Completion. Remove the neck strip and plastic cape. Thoroughly clean all hair clippings from the cape, client's clothing, and the work area. You may then proceed with the next professional service desired by the client.

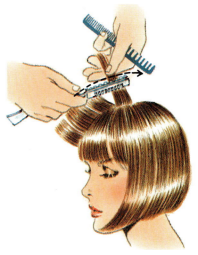

7.49—Shaping section No. 1.

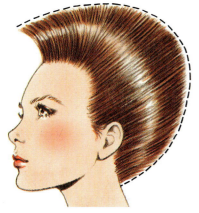

7.50—Correct uniform shaping.

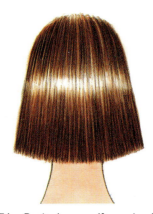

7.51—Back view—uniform shaping.

Question & Answer

LAYERING LONG HAIR

Q: *How much layering should I put in long hair?*

A: It's easy to be confused about "layering" the hair; the word is often misused. Layering simply means making the hair variable lengths throughout an established form.

The confusion comes from misinterpreting the various ways layering can be used to enhance a hairstyle. Most clients associate the word "layering" with shortening the hair to different lengths throughout the entire head. This is not the function of layering.

When the hair is held at 90 degrees (straight away from its natural growth) and cut to a given length throughout, it is considered an all-over layered cut.

Used to enhance long hair, perimeter layers are created by holding the hair at a slight elevation while establishing the hanging length. If you hold the hair flat against the head, no elevation equals no layering. If the hair is held at a 45-degree elevation the perimeter will be moderately layered. This slight perimeter layering will promote softness, remove excess weight and cause the ends to move freely.

Top and crown layering is most common, as it removes some of the length in the crown and the frontal areas so the hair will move away from the head. If the hair is left too long in the crown the hair will lie flat to the head. If the crown hair is cut slightly shorter the hair, with less weight and gravity pull, will stand away from the head, giving the look of volume.

—*From* Milady's Salon Solutions *by Louise Cotter*

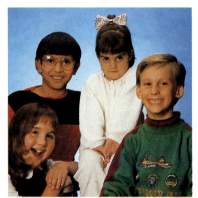

7.52—Popular hairstyles for children.

LEARN TO HANDLE CHILDREN

Special consideration should be given to children and teenagers. Hairstylists who are patient and know how to handle children will attract the parents to their salons for their own hairstyling. (Fig. 7.52)

CUTTING OVERLY CURLY HAIR

Overly curly hair has special characteristics, as have other types of hair, that require certain techniques for styling. Most important to you is the ability to visualize and create a hairstyle that will enhance the appearance of the client. Knowing the correct cutting and styling techniques and using common sense in their application are basic to the success of the hairstylist. One method for shaping and styling overly curly hair is outlined next. Your instructor may also have alternate methods for you to use.

Procedure

1. Drape the client for hair shaping.
2. Shampoo and thoroughly dry the hair.
3. Apply an *emollient* (i-**MOL**-yent) (softening) product lightly to the scalp and hair to replace lost oil.
4. Begin in the crown. Using a wide-tooth comb or a hair lifter, comb the hair upward and slightly forward, extending the hair length as long as possible. Continue until all hair has been combed out from the scalp and evenly distributed around the head. Combing in a circular pattern will usually help avoid splits.
5. Cut the hair. Visualize the style and length of hair desired. Start by tapering the sides, and cut in the direction the hair will be combed.
6. Taper the back part of the head to blend with the sides.
7. Trim the extreme hair ends in the crown and top areas to the desired length.
8. For an off-the-face hairstyle, comb hair up and backward. For a forward movement, comb hair up and forward.
9. Blend side hair with the top, crown, and back hair.
10. Outline the hairstyle at the sides, around the ears, and in the nape area, using either scissors or a trimmer (clipper).
11. Check silhouette of shaping, making sure it is blended.
12. Give a finishing touch. Fluff the hair slightly with a hair lifter, wherever needed. Spray the hair lightly to give it a natural, lustrous sheen. (See Fig. 7.53) ✔

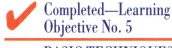
Completed—Learning Objective No. 5

BASIC TECHNIQUES FOR CUTTING WITH SCISSORS OR WITH A RAZOR

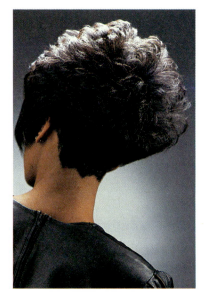
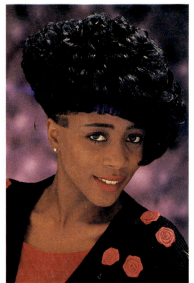
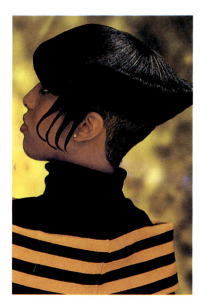

7.53—Popular finished hairstyles.

REVIEW QUESTIONS

HAIRCUTTING

1. Why is the mastery of haircutting so important to the student? *page 84*
2. What four factors should be taken into consideration when choosing a hairstyle for your client? *84*
3. What are the tools used in haircutting? *85*
4. What is the first step in haircutting? *86-87*
5. What is the purpose of thinning the hair? *87*
6. How close to the scalp should you thin: a) fine hair; b) medium hair; c) coarse hair? *page 88*
7. In which areas is it advisable not to thin the hair? *88*
8. Define slithering. *89-90.*
9. What is the purpose of a guideline? *90*
10. What is shingling? *93*
11. For what purpose is the clipper used? *94*
12. Why is a razor used on damp hair? *94*
13. What is tapering? *99*
14. Overly curly hair is cut wet or dry? *98-99.*

FINGER WAVING

8

LEARNING OBJECTIVES

AFTER COMPLETING THIS CHAPTER, YOU SHOULD BE ABLE TO:

1. Explain the purpose of finger waving.
2. Demonstrate the different types of finger waves.
3. List the steps in the finger waving procedure.

INTRODUCTION

Finger waving is the art of shaping and directing the hair into alternate parallel waves and designs using the fingers, comb, waving lotion, and hairpins or clippies.

You may wonder why you are learning a technique that is not frequently requested by many clients anymore. Training in finger waving is important because it teaches you the technique of moving and directing hair. It also helps you develop the dexterity, coordination, and finger strength required for professional hairstyling. In addition, it provides valuable training in creating hairstyles and in molding hair to the curved surface of the head. It is an excellent introduction to hairstyling.

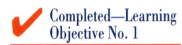

Completed—Learning Objective No. 1

PURPOSE OF FINGER WAVING

PREPARATION

Always wash your hands before giving your client any salon service. Make sure all necessary implements have been sanitized and towels and other supplies are clean and fresh. Prepare the client in the same manner as you would for a shampoo.

Shampoo the client's hair at the shampoo bowl, towel-blot the hair, and seat the client comfortably at your station.

More natural soft-looking waves are obtained with hair that has a natural wave or has been permanently waved than with straight hair. A finger wave correctly done complements the client's head as well as her facial features.

FINGER WAVING LOTION

Waving lotion makes the hair pliable and keeps it in place during the finger waving procedure.

Waving lotion is made from karaya gum, which is found in trees of Africa and India. This gum can be diluted to a thin, watery consistency, generally for use on fine hair, or its consistency can be more concentrated for use on regular or coarse hair. A good waving lotion is harmless to the hair and does not flake when it dries.

APPLICATION OF LOTION

Part the hair down to the scalp, comb smooth, and arrange it to conform to the planned style. The hair will move more easily if you use the coarse teeth of the comb. Follow the natural growth pattern when combing and parting the hair. You will find the hair easier to mold, and it will not buckle or separate in the crown area.

Waving lotion is applied to the hair while it is damp. This permits the lotion to be distributed smoothly and evenly. Use an applicator to apply the waving lotion and a comb to distribute it through the hair. Do not use an excessive amount of waving lotion.

◆ **NOTE:** Apply lotion to one side of the head at a time; this prevents it from drying and requiring additional applications.

To determine the natural hair growth, comb the hair away from the face, and push hair forward gently with the palm of your hand. As you will learn in the chapter on hairstyling, the hair will fall in its natural growth pattern.

The finger wave may be started on either side of the head. However, in this presentation, the hair is parted on the left side of the head and the wave is started on the right (heavy) side of the head.

HORIZONTAL FINGER WAVING

SHAPING THE TOP AREA

Using the index finger of your left hand as a guide, shape the top hair with a comb, using a circular movement. Starting at the hairline, work toward the crown in 1½" to 2" (3.7 to 5 cm) sections at a time until the crown has been reached. (See Fig. 8.1)

Forming the First Ridge

Place the index finger of the left hand directly above the position for the first ridge. With the teeth of the comb pointing slightly upward, insert the comb directly under the index finger. Draw the comb forward about 1" (2.5 cm) along the fingertip. (See Fig. 8.2)

With the teeth still inserted in the ridge, flatten the comb against the head in order to hold the ridge in place. (See Fig. 8.3)

Remove the left hand from the head and place the middle finger above the ridge and the index finger on the teeth of the comb.

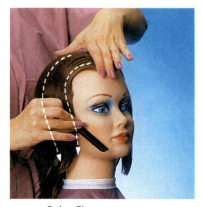

8.1—Shape top area.

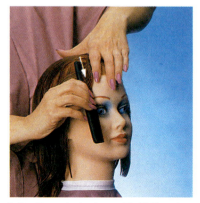

8.2—Draw hair about 1" (2.5 cm) toward fingertip.

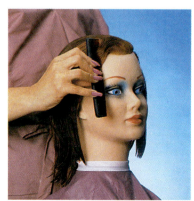

8.3—Flatten comb against head.

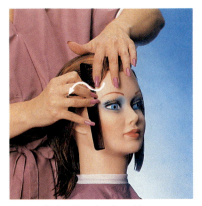

8.4—Emphasize ridge.

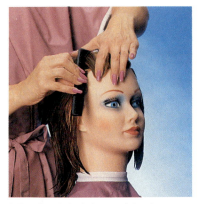

8.5—Comb hair in semicircular direction.

Emphasize the ridge by closing the two fingers and applying pressure to the head. (See Fig. 8.4)

◆ **NOTE:** Do not try to increase the height or depth of a ridge by pinching or pushing with fingers; such movements will create over-direction of the ridge.

Without removing the comb, turn the teeth downward, and comb the hair in a right semicircular direction to form a dip in the hollow part of the wave. (See Fig. 8.5)

Follow this procedure, section by section, until the crown has been reached, where the ridge phases out. (See Fig. 8.6)

The ridge and wave of each section should match evenly, without showing separations in the ridge and hollow part of the wave.

Forming the Second Ridge

Begin at the crown area. (See Fig. 8.7) The movements are the reverse of those followed in forming the first ridge. The comb is drawn from the tip of the index finger toward the base of the index finger, thus directing formation of the second ridge. All movements are followed in a reverse pattern until the hairline is reached, thus completing the second ridge. (See Fig. 8.8)

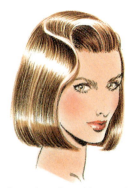

8.6—Complete first ridge at the crown.

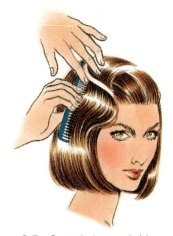

8.7—Start the second ridge.

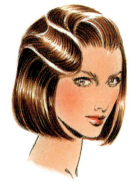

8.8—Complete second ridge.

Forming the Third Ridge

Movements for the third ridge closely follow those used in creating the first ridge. However, the third ridge is started at the hairline and extended back toward the back of the head. (See Fig. 8.9)

Continue alternating directions until the side of the head has been completed. (See Fig. 8.10)

CHAPTER 8   FINGER WAVING   ◆   105

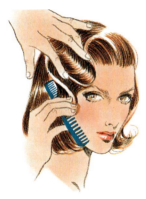

8.9—Start the third ridge.

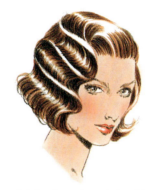

8.10—Complete right side.

LEFT SIDE OF THE HEAD

Use the same procedure for the left (light) side of the head as you used for finger waving the right (heavy) side of the head.

Procedure

1. Shape the hair. (See Fig. 8.11)
2. Starting at the hairline, form the first ridge, section by section, until the second ridge of the opposite side is reached. (See Fig. 8.12)
3. Both the ridge and the wave must blend without splits or breaks, with the ridge and wave on the right side of the head. (See Fig. 8.13)
4. Start with the ridge and wave in the back of the head and proceed, section by section, toward the left side of the face.
5. Continue working back and forth until the entire side is completed. (See Fig. 8.14)

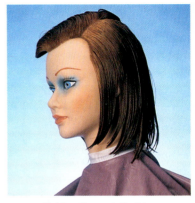

8.11—Shape left side.

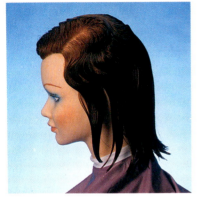

8.12—First ridge starts at hairline.

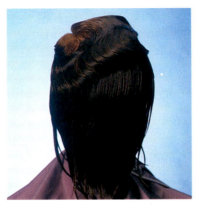

8.13—Ridge and wave matched in the crown area.

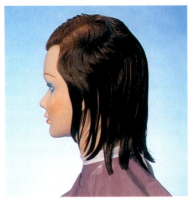

8.14—Left side completed.

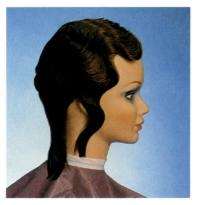
8.15—Completed hairstyle, right side.

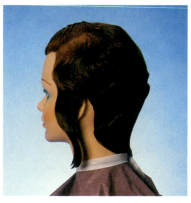
8.16—Completed hairstyle, left side.

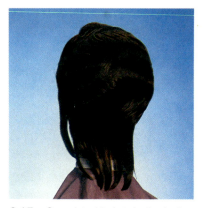
8.17—Completed hairstyle, back view.

6. Figures 8.15–8.17 illustrate the completed hairstyles.

Completion

1. Place net over hair, secure with hairpins or clippies if needed, and safeguard the client's forehead and ears while under the dryer with cotton, gauze, or paper protectors.
2. Adjust the dryer to medium heat and allow hair to dry thoroughly.
3. Remove client from under dryer.
4. Remove clippies or pins and hairnet from hair.
5. Comb out and reset waves into a soft coiffure.
6. Clean up workstation.
7. Sanitize combs, hairpins, clippies, and hairnet after each use.

ALTERNATE METHOD OF FINGER WAVING

Hair parted on left side. The following is an alternate method to perform finger waving:

1. Shape the top right (heavy) side.
2. Phase out the first ridge starting at the front *right* side, and working around to the crown.
3. Start a ridge on the *left* front side and go all around the head, finishing on the front right hairline. (Fig. 8.18)
4. Start another ridge on the front right hairline and finish on the left front side. Continue, left to right and right to left, until the entire head is completed.

This method eliminates the need to match ridges and waves at the back of the head. (Completion is the same as it is for the horizontal method of finger waving.)

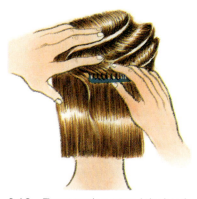
8.18—Finger waving around the head.

VERTICAL FINGER WAVING

In vertical finger waving, the ridges and waves run up and down the head, while in horizontal finger waving they go parallel around the head.

The procedure for making vertical ridges and waves is the same as it is for horizontal finger waving.

1. Make side part, extending from forehead to crown.
2. Form shaping in a semicircular effect. (See Figs. 8.19, 8.20)

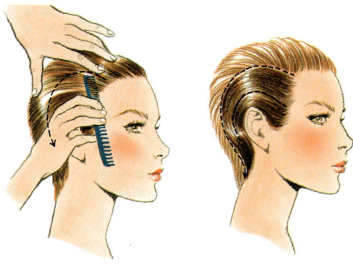

8.19—Form shaping.   8.20—First section of wave.

3. Make first section of ridge and wave. (See Fig. 8.21)
4. Continue with additional sections until the part is reached.

Start the second ridge at the hair part. Start the third ridge at the hairline. Complete side. (See Fig. 8.22) (Completion is the same as it is for horizontal finger waving.)

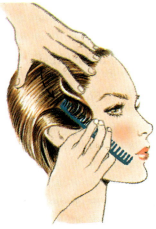
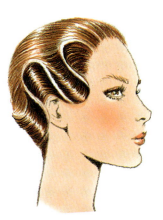

8.21—Start first wave.   8.22—Completed finger wave.

SHADOW WAVE

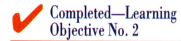
Completed—Learning Objective No. 2

DIFFERENT TYPES OF FINGER WAVES

A shadow wave is a shallow wave with low ridges that are not very sharp. The waves are formed in the regular manner, but the comb does not penetrate to the scalp. The hair layers underneath are not waved. This type of wave is sometimes desirable for a client who wishes to dress her hair very close to the head.

REMINDERS AND HINTS ON FINGER WAVING

1. Wash hands and have available sanitized implements and supplies.
2. Avoid the use of an excessive amount of waving lotion.
3. Use hard rubber combs with both fine and coarse teeth.
4. Before finger waving, locate the natural or permanent wave in the hair.
5. To emphasize the ridges of a finger wave, press the ridge between the fingers, holding the fingers against the head.
6. To wave the underneath hair, insert the comb through the hair to the scalp.
7. For a longer-lasting finger wave, mold the waves in the direction of the natural growth.
8. To safeguard the client's forehead and ears from intense heat while under dryer, use cotton, gauze, or paper protectors.
9. Place a net over the hair to protect the setting while it is being dried.
10. Thoroughly dry the hair before combing it out.
11. Prolonged drying under heat will dry the natural oils of the hair and scalp.
12. Finger waves will not remain in place if the hair is combed out before it has been completely dried.
13. Lightened or tinted hair that tangles is easier to comb if a cream rinse is used.
14. Lightly spraying the hair with lacquer will hold the finger wave longer and give the hair a sheen.

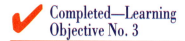
Completed—Learning Objective No. 3

STEPS IN FINGER WAVING PROCEDURES

Promo Power

TELEMARKETING

Telemarketing can be done from within your salon any time someone is available to spend time talking on the phone with your clients—or you can hire an outside person to do telephone soliciting for you. Either way, this kind of advertising has its advantages: It's a personal, one-on-one communication and you get instant results.

To use telemarketing effectively you must be clear about what you want to accomplish. You may want to ask a new client how the service was, how the style was, whether he or she is planning to return. This type of information can be solicited easily by a staff member.

If you're trying to mass-market your salon, you'll want to hire a telemarketing company. You must tell them what you're promoting and give them a script to use. You may want to do a survey on why customers have not returned to your salon or whether your services are satisfactory.

Telemarketing can be very beneficial, but you must have computerized telephone lists in order to do it efficiently. Keep careful records on your own clients. It you are looking for new customers, you can buy telephone lists categorized according to lifestyle, income, or geographical area. Make sure you market to people who would fit in with your type of salon.

—*From* The Salon Biz: Tips for Success *by Geri Mataya*

REVIEW QUESTIONS

FINGER WAVING

1. What is the purpose of finger waving? *page 102*
2. What is the purpose of finger waving lotion? *102*
3. Name the different types of finger waves. *103, 106, 107 & 108*
4. List five reminders or hints for better finger waving. *108*

WET HAIRSTYLING

9

LEARNING OBJECTIVES

AFTER COMPLETING THIS CHAPTER, YOU SHOULD BE ABLE TO:

1. Define hairstyling.
2. List the basic elements of pin curl hairstyling.
3. Demonstrate the procedures and the proper use and care of implements employed in hairstyling.
4. List and analyze the characteristics of a client's appearance prior to a hairstyling service.

INTRODUCTION

Before you can become a proficient stylist you must first understand hair structure, permanent waving, hair straightening, thermal waving and curling, hair coloring, hair chemistry, the action of conditioners, and the overall importance of hair shaping.

Hairstyling is creating wearable art. To be a successful stylist you must be able to apply basic art principles to hairstyling in order to change along with fashion trends.

The elementary rules of art that you use to style hair are weight and balance, form, rhythm, shape, composition, contrast, elevation, texture, structure, and the use of space. The accomplishments of styling, decoration, and incorporating new ideas become easier as you gain experience.

As you gain experience you will become adept at using art principles and applying them appropriately to each client. It is advisable for you to take note of your client's physical form so that you will be better able to balance the hairstyle to the individual.

Examine your client's hair before starting the shampoo. This gives you the opportunity to take note of hair growth direction and texture, determine which implements to use, and helps you visualize a becoming and personalized hairstyle. (Fig. 9.1)

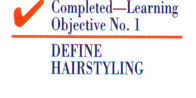

✓ Completed—Learning Objective No. 1

DEFINE HAIRSTYLING

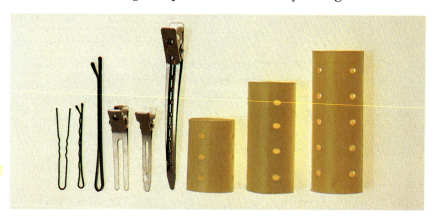

9.1—Implements and materials used in hairstyling—left to right: hairpin; bobby pin; roller pin; double prong clip (clippie); single prong clip (clippie); duckbill clamp (clippie); short roller; medium roller; long roller.

HAIRSTYLING BASICS

REMOVING TANGLES FROM HAIR

It is necessary to remove tangles from your client's hair before you shampoo, cut, or style it. This will prevent damage and matting. To remove tangles, follow this procedure:

1. Begin at the nape with a coarse-toothed comb or cushioned brush.
2. Separate a small section and brush across and down each strand.
3. Work across the back, in small sections, gradually progressing to the crown.
4. The size of the sections you use will depend on the thickness, length, curliness, condition, and elasticity of the hair.

5. Once the tangles are removed, proceed with the service. (Figs. 9.2–9.4)

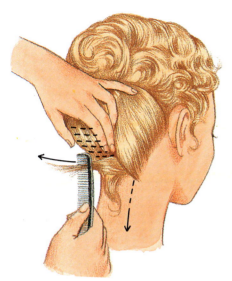
9.2—Removing tangles in nape area.

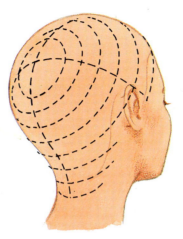
9.3—Combing pattern for removing tangles.

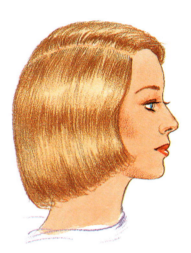
9.4—Tangles removed.

MAKING A PART

Clean partings make hairstyles look professional. Use any one of these common methods.

1. Comb hair straight and tightly back from the face. Draw your comb toward the back of the head in an even line. Hold the light side firm while combing the heavy side away from the parting. (Figs. 9.5–9.7)
2. Using the end of a tail comb, draw a clean, clear line.
3. To make use of a *natural part,* comb wet hair straight back. Place the palm of the left hand on the head and push forward. You will notice the hair split apart into sections. These sections are the natural partings.

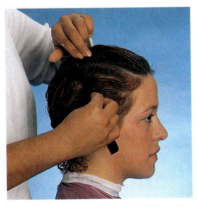
9.5—Drawing comb back full length.

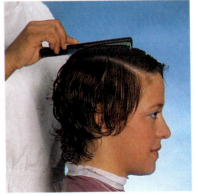
9.6—Combing hair above and below part.

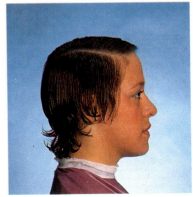
9.7—Hair combed with straight part.

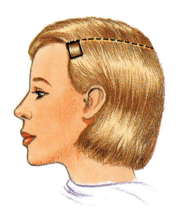

9.8—Parts of a curl.

PIN CURLS

Pin curls provide the bases for all patterns, lines, waves, curls, and rolls that you use as you create hairstyles. You can use them on straight, permanent-waved, and naturally curly hair. Pin curls work best if the hair is properly tapered and wound smoothly. This makes springy and long-lasting curls with good direction and definition.

Parts of a Curl

Pin curls are constructed of three principal parts: *base*, *stem*, and *circle*. (Fig. 9.8)

1. The **base** is the stationary, or immovable, foundation of the curl, which is attached to the scalp. (Fig. 9.9)
2. The **stem** is the section of the pin curl, between the base and first arc (turn) of the circle, which gives the circle its direction, action, and mobility.
3. The **circle** is the part of the pin curl that forms a complete circle. The size of the curl governs the width of the wave and its strength.

Mobility of a Curl

The amount of movement (mobility) of a section of hair is determined by the *stem* and *circle*. Curl mobility is classified as *no-stem*, *half-stem*, and *full-stem*.

1. The **no-stem curl** is placed directly on the base of the curl. It produces a tight, firm, long-lasting curl.
2. The **half-stem curl** permits more freedom, since the curl (circle) is placed one-half off the base. It gives good *control* to the hair and produces *softness* in the finished wave pattern.
3. The **full-stem curl** allows for the greatest mobility. The curl is placed completely off the base. The base may be a square, triangular, half-moon, or rectangular section depending on the area of the head in which the full-stem curls are used. It gives as much freedom as the length of the stem will permit. If it is exaggerated, the hair near the scalp will be flat and almost straight. It is used for a *strong direction* of the hair and a *weaker wave pattern*. (Figs. 9.10–9.12)

9.9—Pin curl base.

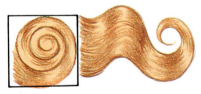

9.10—No-stem curl opened out.

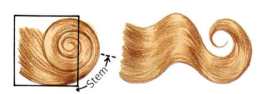

9.11—Half-stem curl opened out.

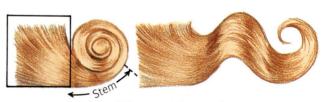

9.12—Full-stem curl opened out.

Open and Closed Center Curls

Open center curls produce even, smooth waves and uniform curls. *Closed center curls* produce waves that decrease in size toward the end. They are good for fine hair or if a fluffy curl is desired. Notice the difference in the waves produced by pin curls with open centers and those with closed centers. The size of the curl determines the size of the wave. If you make pin curls with the ends outside the curl, the resulting wave will be narrower near the scalp and wider toward the ends. (Figs. 9.13, 9.14)

Curl and Stem Direction

Curls may be turned toward the face, away from the face, upward, downward, or diagonally. You determine what the finished result will be by the direction in which you place the stem of the curl. Curl and stem direction is referred to as:

1. *Forward movement*—toward the face.
2. *Reverse movement*—backward or away from the face. (Figs. 9.15–9.18)

These illustrations are intended to show stem directions and curl placements and are not illustrations of pin curl patterns.

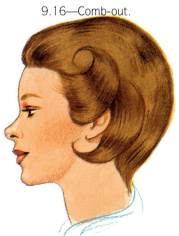

9.13—Curl with open center. 9.14—Curl with closed center.

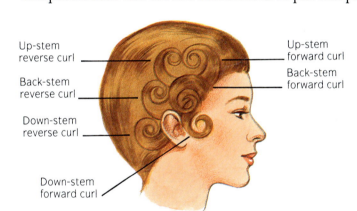

9.15—Forward movement.

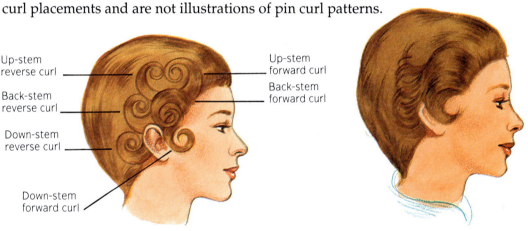

9.16—Comb-out.

9.17—Backward movement.

9.18—Comb-out.

Clockwise and Counterclockwise Curls

The terms *clockwise curls* and *counterclockwise curls* are used to describe the direction of pin curls. Curls formed in the same direction as the movement of the hands of a clock are known as clockwise curls. Curls formed in the opposite direction of the movement of the hands of a clock are known as counterclockwise curls. (Figs. 9.19, 9.20)

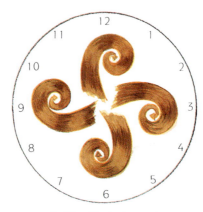

9.19—Clockwise curls.

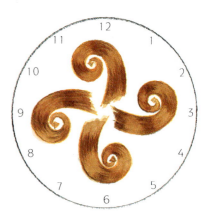

9.20—Counterclockwise curls.

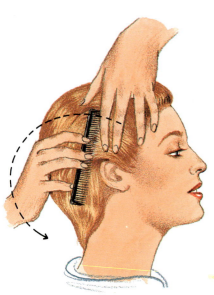

9.21—Forming side forward vertical shaping.

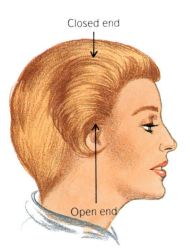

9.22—Finished side forward vertical shaping.

Shaping for Pin Curl Placements

A *shaping* is a section of hair that you mold into a design to serve as a base for a curl or wave pattern.

Shapings are classified as forward and reverse; diagonal, vertical, or horizontal; oblong or circular.

Circular shapings are pie-shaped with the open end smaller than the closed end. They work well as the first forward shaping in a hairstyle that moves away from the face. In a wave pattern, the forward circular shaping would be followed by a reverse circular curl.

Oblong shapings are waves that remain the same width throughout the shaping.

Forward shapings are directed toward the face. This type of shaping is *oval* (larger in size at its closed end).

Procedure

1. To make a forward, vertical shaping on the side of the head, direct the hair in a circular motion, moving back from the face, upward, then downward and toward the face. The size of the shaping determines the resulting hairstyle. (Figs. 9.21, 9.22)

2. To make a top forward shaping, comb-direct the hair in a circular motion, away from the forehead, pivoting the comb to create a circular effect toward the face. (Figs. 9.23, 9.24)

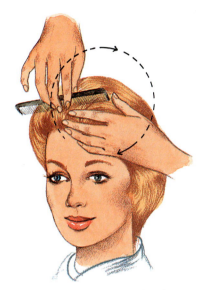
9.23—Forming oval shaping for top forward movement.

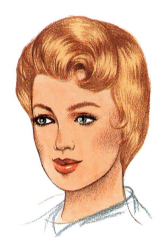
9.24—Finished oval shaping for top forward movement.

Reverse shapings are comb-directed downward, then immediately upward in a circular motion, away from the face. (Figs. 9.25, 9.26)

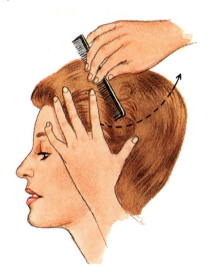
9.25—Forming left side reverse vertical shaping.

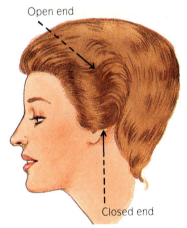
9.26—Finished left side reverse vertical shaping.

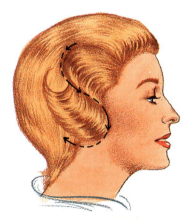
9.27—Diagonal shaping.

Diagonal shapings are variations of the forward shaping with the exception that the shaping is formed diagonally to the side of the head. (Fig. 9.27)

Vertical side shapings are directed in a way that places the open and closed ends in a vertical fashion.

Horizontal shapings are comb-directed parallel with the parting. They are recommended for pin curl parallel construction and where a wave design is carried completely around the head. (Figs. 9.28, 9.29)

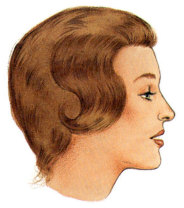 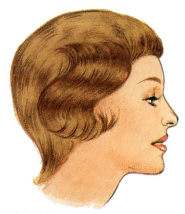

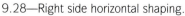

9.28—Right side horizontal shaping.

9.29—Right side reverse horizontal shaping.

PIN CURL FOUNDATIONS OR BASES

Before you begin to make your pin curls, divide the hair into sections or panels. Then you are ready to subdivide the sections into the type of foundations or bases required for the various curls. The most commonly shaped bases you will use are rectangular, triangular, arc (half-moon or C-shape), and square. (Figs. 9.30, 9.31)

To avoid splits in the finished hairstyle, you must use care when selecting and forming the curl base. Further uniformity of curl development can only be achieved if the sections of hair are as equal as possible. Each curl must lie flat and smooth on its base. If extended too far off the base you will get just direction with a loose curl away from the scalp. The finished curl, however, is not affected by the shape of the base.

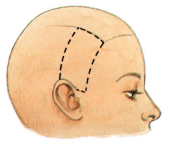 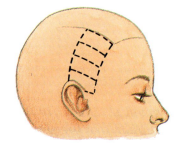

9.30—Panel.

9.31—Panel with rectangular bases.

Rectangular base pin curls are usually recommended at the side front hairline for a smooth upsweep effect. To avoid splits in the comb-out, the pin curls must overlap. (Fig. 9.32)

Triangular base pin curls are recommended along the front or facial hairline to prevent breaks or splits in the finished hairstyle. The triangular base allows a portion of the hair from each curl to overlap the next and comb into a uniform wave without splits. (Figs. 9.33, 9.34)

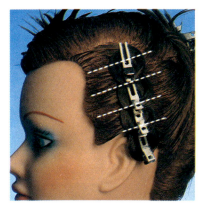 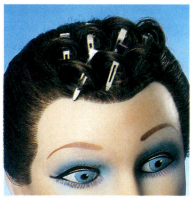 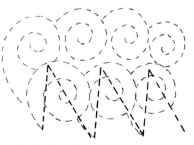

9.32—Rectangular base.   9.33—Triangular base.   9.34—Detail of triangular base.

Arc base, also known as half-moon or C-shape base, pin curls are carved out of a shaping. Arc base pin curls give good direction and may be used for an upsweep effect or a French twist at the lower back of the head. (Figs. 9.35, 9.36)

Square base pin curls are used for even construction suitable for curly hairstyles without much volume or lift. They can be used on any part of the head and will comb out with lasting results. To avoid splits in the comb-out, stagger the sectioning as shown in the illustration (square base, brick-lay fashion). (Fig. 9.37)

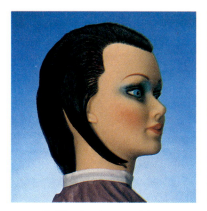 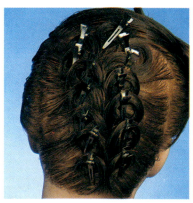 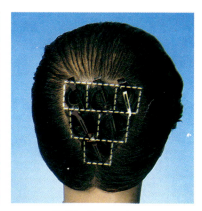

9.35—Arc base—side.   9.36—Arc base—back of head.   9.37—Square base.

PIN CURL TECHNIQUES

You will learn to make pin curls several ways. We illustrate several methods of forming pin curls. Your instructor might demonstrate other methods that are equally correct.

Carved Curls or Sculptured Curls

Pin curls, carved out of a shaping without disturbing the shaping, are usually referred to as *carved curls.* You can form these curls on either the right side or the left side of the head.

Procedure for Forming Pin Curls on the Right Side

1. Wet hair thoroughly with water or setting lotion.
2. Comb smoothly and form shaping. (See Fig. 9.38)
3. Start making curls at the open end of the shaping.
4. Slice strand for first curl. (See Fig. 9.39) Use your finger to hold the curl in place.
5. **Ribbon** the strand by forcing it through the comb while applying pressure with the thumb on the back of comb to create tension. (See Figs. 9.40, 9.41)

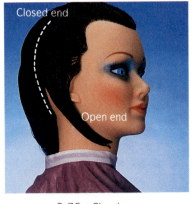

9.38—Shaping.

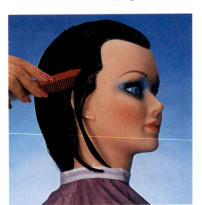

9.39—Slicing.

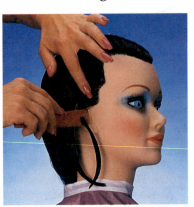

9.40—Holding base with finger.

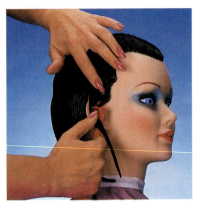

9.41—Ribboning.

6. Form the curl forward. (See Fig. 9.42)
7. Wind the curl around your index finger. (See Fig. 9.43)

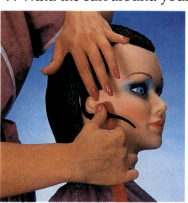

9.42—Forming.

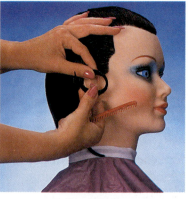

9.43—Winding.

8. Slide the curl off your finger, keeping the hair ends inside the center of the curl. (See Fig. 9.44)
9. Mold the curl into the shaping. (See Fig. 9.45)
10. Hold the curl in shaping. (See Fig. 9.46)
11. Anchor the curl with clip. (See Fig. 9.47)

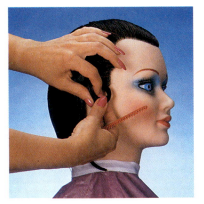
9.44—Sliding off finger.

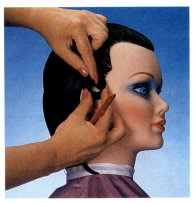
9.45—Molding.

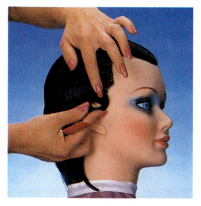
9.46—Holding curl.

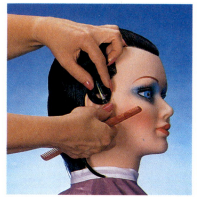
9.47—Anchoring.

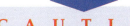

CAUTION
Be very careful not to destroy your shaping as you comb or pin the curl.

Whenever a longer-lasting curl movement is desired, stretch the hair strand and apply tension. You can accomplish this by ribboning and stretching the strand. Firmly comb it between the spine of the comb and the thumb in the direction of the curl movement.

Sculptured curl arrangements backed up with a second row of pin curls comb out into strong ridge waves. (Figs. 9.48–9.50)

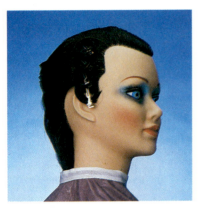

9.48—Finished first row.

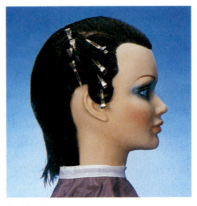

9.49—Sculpture curl arrangement backed up with a second row of curls.

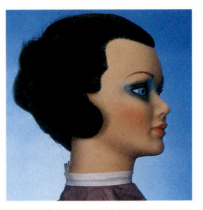

9.50—Curls combed into waves with a strong ridge.

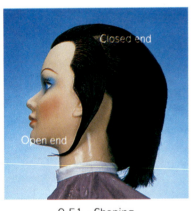

9.51—Shaping.

Procedure for Forming Pin Curls on the Left Side

Making pin curls on the left side of the head requires a different technique from making them on the right side.

1. Wet hair thoroughly with water or setting lotion. Comb smooth and form the shaping. (See Fig. 9.51) Note open and closed ends of shaping.
2. Slice a strand out of shaping. (See Fig. 9.52)
3. Stretch a strand by ribboning it through the comb. (See Figs. 9.53, 9.54)

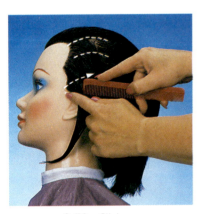

9.52—Slicing.

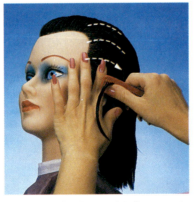

9.53—Holding base with finger and stretching strand by pulling through the comb.

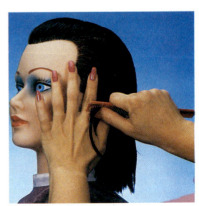

9.54—Ribboning.

4. Form a forward curl.
5. Wind the strand around your index finger. (See Fig. 9.55)
6. Slide the curl off tip of your finger and mold into shaping. (See Fig. 9.56)
7. Hold the curl in shaping. (See Fig. 9.57)
8. Anchor with a clip. (See Fig. 9.58)

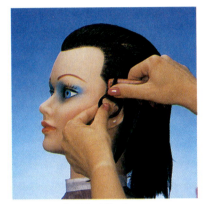
9.55—Winding.

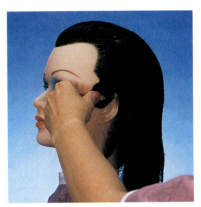
9.56—Sliding off finger.

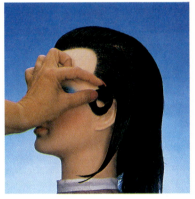
9.57—Holding curl.

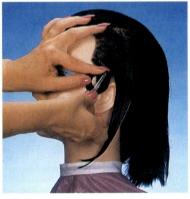
9.58—Anchoring.

What You Should Know about Pin Curls

1. Pin curls must fit within the curvature of a shaping. (See Fig. 9.59)
2. Curls should overlap one another.
3. The size of the curls graduates from small at the open end to large at the closed end.

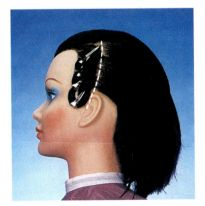
9.59—Finished first row.

4. Reverse shaping for backup curls. (See Fig. 9.60)
5. To slice a strand, the tip of your comb should touch the tip of your finger halfway through shaping. (See Fig. 9.61)

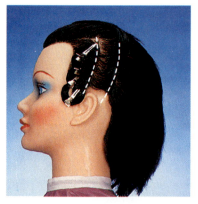
9.60—Reverse shaping.

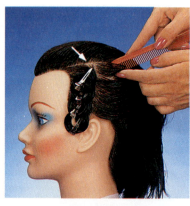
9.61—Slicing.

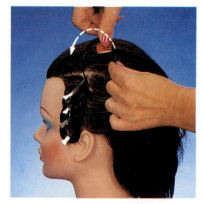
9.62—Ribboning.

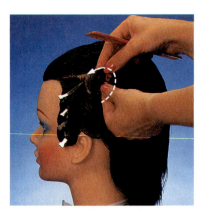
9.63—Placing curl.

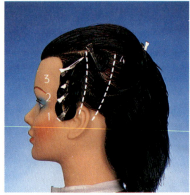
9.64—Completed first curl.

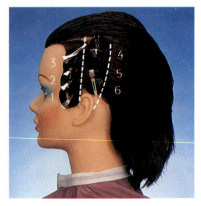
9.65—Completed reverse shaping.

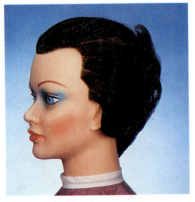
9.66—Comb-out.

6. To ribbon hair you will use the coarse or fine teeth of the comb depending on the hair texture. (See Fig. 9.62)
7. Ribbon the tip of the strand with fine teeth for a neat closing of the curl and place on base. (See Fig. 9.63)
8. Complete top reverse curl and divide shaping into strands for the next two curls. (See Fig. 9.64)
9. Complete the second row of curls within the curve of the shaping. (See Fig. 9.65)
10. Comb out the forward and reverse pin curl setting into a full, wide wave. (See Fig. 9.66)

ANCHORING PIN CURLS

Anchoring pin curls correctly ensures that curls hold firmly where you have placed them, so that the hairstyle you have planned develops properly.

There are several methods for inserting clips or clippies, but they are always inserted from the *open* end of the shaping. Whichever way you choose, keep in mind that it is essential not to disturb the base or sculpture as you insert the clip.

Procedure

To anchor the pin curl correctly, gently slide the clip or clippie through part of the base and/or stem at an angle and across the ends of the curl. This will hold the curl securely without it unfurling, sagging, or flipping over.

1. Clips should be anchored in such a manner that they do not interfere with the formation or placement of other curls or with any other step in setting the hair.

2. To avoid indentation or impressions across the hair, it is advisable not to pin across the center of the entire curl.

3. The size of the clips used should be governed by the size of the curl. Curls made with small strands or fine hair cannot support the weight of a double-prong clip, but perform better if pinned in place with a single-prong clip (clippie) or hairpin. However, a clippie or hairpin might not be able to support the weight of coarse or thick hair. Use your own judgment.

4. Clips that are placed against the skin, ear, or scalp can become very hot during the drying process. If clips must touch the skin, simply place cotton under the part of the clips touching these areas. (Figs. 9.67–9.70)

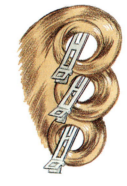

9.67—Hairline forward pin curls (clockwise curl).

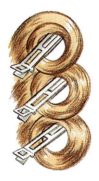

9.68—Forward pin curls equal in size. Any place on the head.

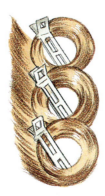

9.69—Reverse pin curls (counterclockwise curls). Equal in size. Any place on the head.

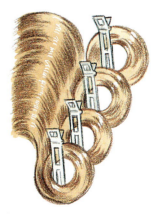

9.70—Ridge reverse pin curls (counterclockwise curls).

EFFECTS OF PIN CURLS

Pin curl patterns have been designed to achieve specific style effects. Always take care to ensure that pin curls lie evenly and are placed in the direction in which they will be combed; otherwise, you will find yourself fighting uneven wave or curl design.

1. A *vertical wave* produces the best result when it begins with a reverse shaping, followed by a pin curl pattern. (Figs. 9.71, 9.72)

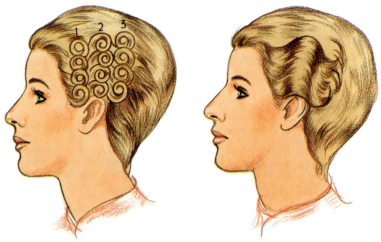

9.71—Vertical wave pin curl pattern.   9.72—Vertical wave comb-out.

2. A *horizontal wave* is first shaped in a forward semicircular fashion, from the hair part downward. The pin curls are then set. (Figs. 9.73, 9.74)

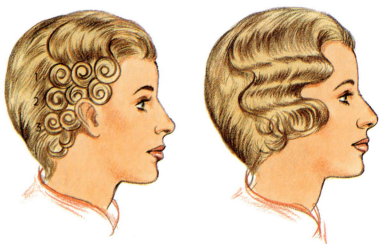

9.73—Horizontal wave pin curl pattern.   9.74—Horizontal wave comb-out.

3. *Interlocking movement* involves two directional rows of pin curls and produces clash (an area where two wave patterns are placed back to back to build volume). First row—back stem with forward curls. Second row—forward stem with

reverse curls. Comb-out—the clash area is interlocked. (Figs. 9.75, 9.76)

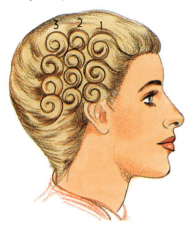
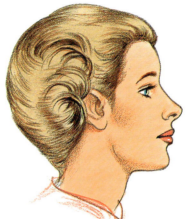

9.75—Setting pattern.   9.76—Comb-out.

4. *Waved top.* (Figs. 9.77–9.79)

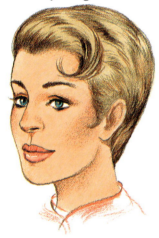
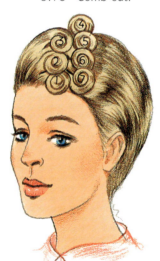
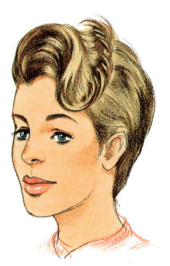

9.77—Shaping.   9.78—Setting pattern.   9.79—Comb-out.

5. *Diagonal waves* are made by shaping hair in an oval forward. Then start the pin curls at the open end. (Figs. 9.80, 9.81)

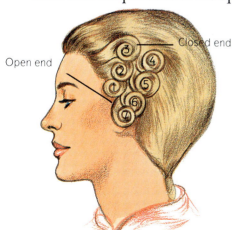
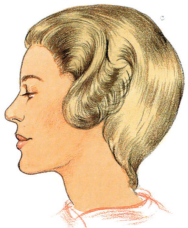

9.80—Setting pattern.   9.81—Comb-out.

6. For *waved bangs,* shape the hair and set the pin curls into waves starting at the open end. For fine hair use more pin curls than you would for normal hair. (Figs. 9.82–9.85)

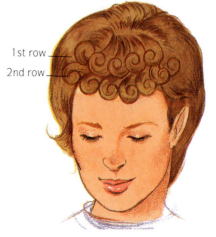
9.82—Setting pattern for fine hair.

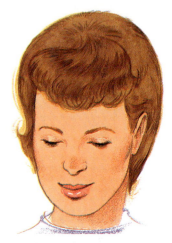
9.83—Comb-out.

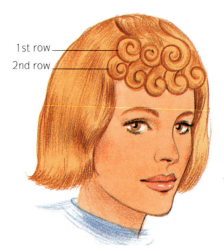
9.84—Setting pattern for normal hair.

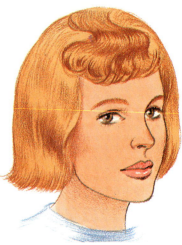
9.85—Comb-out.

7. A *French twist* is set by parting off the back area and making a vertical center part. Comb both sections together, as they will be in the finished comb-out. Shape large, smooth pin curls into the two long vertical shapings. Comb out by back-brushing or back-combing the area. Smooth one side with a narrow brush, and pin the ends down with a row of bobby pins. Smooth the other section, and fold the ends over the first hair in herringbone fashion. Tuck the ends in, and pin with a neat row of bobby pins. (Figs. 9.86, 9.87)

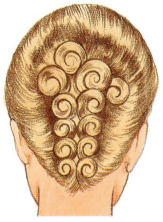

9.86—Setting pattern for normal hair.

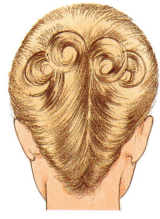

9.87—Comb-out and pinning.

8. ***Ridge curls*** are pin curls placed behind the ridge of a shaping or finger wave. They are useful when a loose wave with good definition is desired. You must be careful not to disturb the ridge when slicing out the strands for the curls. (Figs. 9.88–9.91)

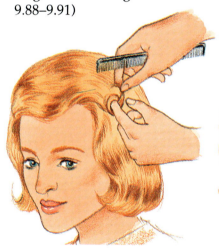

9.88—Wind hair around fingertip.

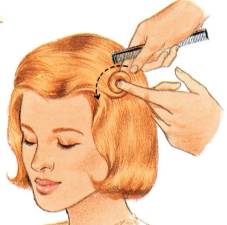

9.89—Slide strand off finger and roll it to base of ridge.

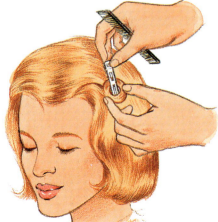

9.90—Anchor curl with clippie.

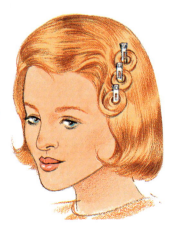

9.91—Completed ridge curl.

✓ Completed—Learning Objective No. 2

BASIC PIN CURL HAIRSTYLING

9. *Skip waves* are formed by a combination of finger waves and pin curl patterns. The pin curls are placed in *alternate* finger wave formations. This technique is recommended when side, smooth-flowing vertical waves are desired. For best results the hair should be 3" to 5" (7.5 to 12.5 cm) in length. (Figs. 9.92–9.94) It is not suitable for very curly or fine hair. ✓

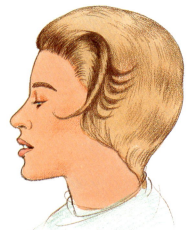

9.92—Shaping and ridge for vertical finger wave.

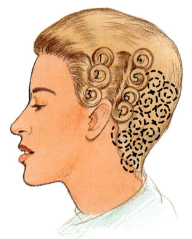

9.93—Skip wave pattern for fluff ends.

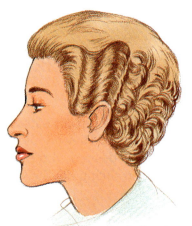

9.94—Comb-out with fluff ends.

CASCADE OR STAND UP CURLS

The *cascade or stand up curl* is the forerunner of the roller. It provides for height in the finished hairstyle and may be used with rollers or alone. It is wound from the ends to the scalp, as a roller is. The center opening is made large, and the curl is pinned in a standing position. (Figs. 9.95–9.102)

Procedure

Wet hair thoroughly with water or setting lotion.

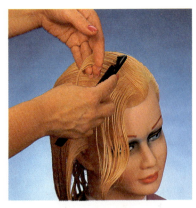

9.95—Comb, divide, and smooth strand.

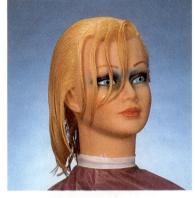

9.96—Divide the section into strands for individual curls.

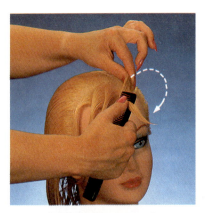

9.97—Ribbon strand.

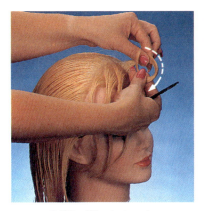
9.98—Direct strand.

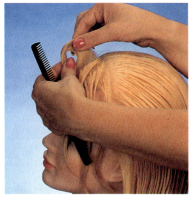
9.99—Wind the strand, being sure to keep the curl round.

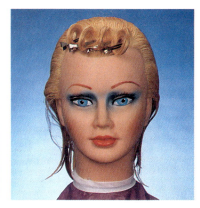
9.100—Anchor the curl securely at the base.

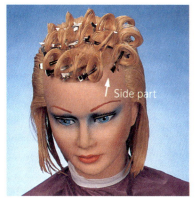
9.101—Top setting.

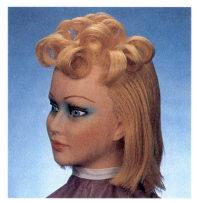
9.102—Comb out as you would a roller set.

SEMI-STAND UP CURLS

Semi-stand up curls are stand up curls that have been carved out of a shaping and pinned in a semi-standing position. A top wave effect can be achieved with semi-stand up curls. After the shaping is in place, make three counterclockwise curls, and back them up with four clockwise curls. (Figs. 9.103–9.105)

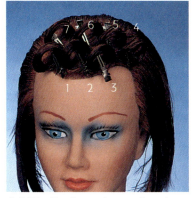
9.103—Semi-stand up curl setting.

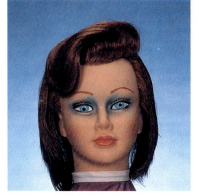
9.104—Comb-out.

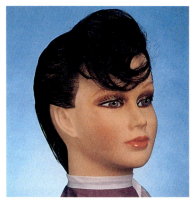
9.105—(Alternate) Comb-out.

ROLLER CURLS

You can use rollers to create the same effects as stand up curls. They are simply molds for stand up curls, which allow you to have more control over the hair. Like stand up curls, they create a great deal of lift and volume. There are advantages to using roller curls rather than pin curl methods.

1. One roller can accommodate the equivalent of two to four stand up curls.
2. Rollers give more security to hair when it is wet, so there is no chance of having your finely executed curls collapse.
3. The tension with which hair can be placed on a roller gives the finished curl a bounce and life that a pin curl cannot provide.
4. Rollers come in various sizes, lengths, and shapes to fulfill most hairstyling needs. (Fig. 9.106)

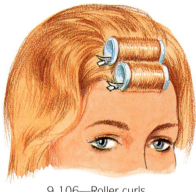

9.106—Roller curls.

Roller Technique

1. Section hair into panels, then subdivide each panel into roller bases.
2. The size of the base should be almost the same size as the roller. If a roller is 3" (7.5 cm) long and 1" (2.5 cm) wide, the base for it should be 2½" (6.25 cm) long and 1" (2.5 cm) wide. The size of the base will be guided by the size of the roller.
3. Hair must be wet so that it will be flexible, stretchable, and adhere to plastic rollers.
4. Prepare a roller section by combing the strand firmly and smoothly at a 45° (.785 rad.) angle. (See Figs. 9.107, 9.108a–b)
5. Wrap ends of the hair smoothly against the roller.

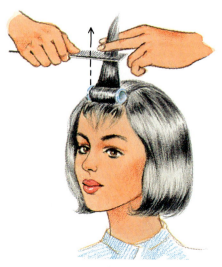

9.107—Strand preparation.

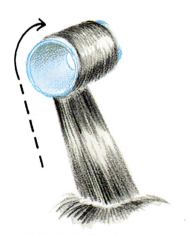

9.108a—45° angle.

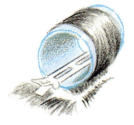

9.108b—Anchor with clip.

6. Place both thumbs over the hair ends and roll the roller firmly toward the scalp. (See Figs. 9.109, 9.110)

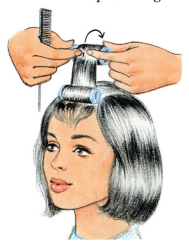

9.109—Winding roller.

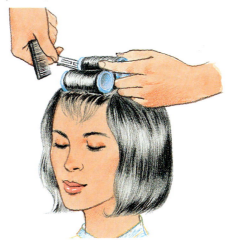

9.110—Pinning roller.

7. Hold the roller in position while clipping. (See Figs. 9.111–9.114)

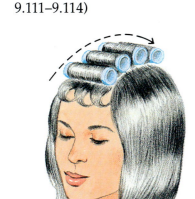

9.111—Complete panel of roller curls from hairline to crown with strands left out for bang effect.

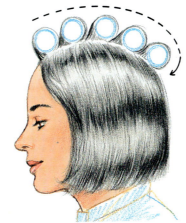

9.112—Roller setting for off-the-face effect.

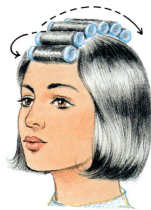

9.113—Roller curl pattern for bang effect.

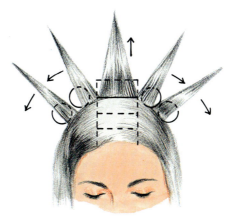

9.114—The angle at which hair should be held from the head for roller placement.

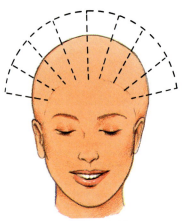

9.115—Sectioning of different lengths of hair for rollers.

Roller Size

Rollers are most effective in creating lift and volume, and indentation (valleys and hollows) in hairstyles.

◆**NOTE:** To use rollers to their best advantage, it is important for the hair length to be more than three times the rollers' diameter. For example, a roller with a 1½" (3.75 cm) diameter is for use on hair that is 4½" (11.25 cm) long. (Fig. 9.115)

A strand of hair that is 4½" (11.25 cm) long will wrap around a 1" (2.5 cm) roller one full turn. The result will be a soft puff with minimum curl on the ends. (Figs. 9.116, 9.117)

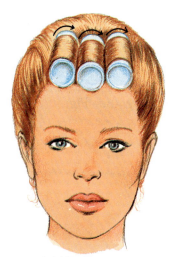
9.116—Pattern.

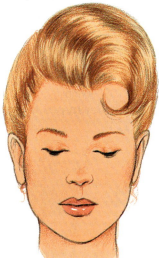
9.117—Comb-out.

When using a ¾" (1.85 cm) roller on hair that is 4½" (11.25 cm) long, the strand will wrap around 1½ times. The result will be a curlier set. (Figs. 9.118, 9.119)

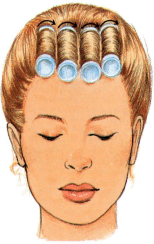
9.118—Pattern.

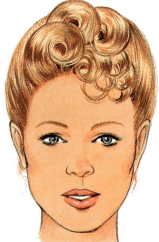
9.119—Comb-out.

One-half-inch (1.25 cm) rollers permit the hair to wrap around two or more times, resulting in a deep, soft wave with clash. (The hair ends turn in the opposite direction from the movement.) Notice that you need more rollers to cover the same area. (Figs. 9.120, 9.121)

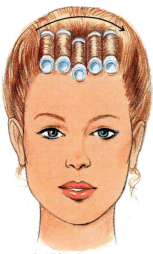 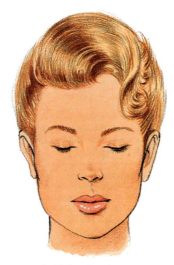

9.120—Pattern.   9.121—Comb-out.

◆ **NOTE:** The length of the hair and size of the roller affect the finished hairstyle. If you use a roller that is 1½" (3.75 cm) in diameter on hair that is 6" to 7" (15 to 17.5 cm) long, you will get different results than you would with hair that is 3" to 5" (7.5 to 12.5 cm) in length.

BARREL CURLS

A barrel curl serves as a substitute for a curl formed around a roller. It may be used where there is insufficient room to place a roller. However, it does not provide the tension that is present in roller wrapping.

The barrel curl is made in a similar manner as the stand up curl, with a flat base and containing much more hair. (Fig. 9.122)

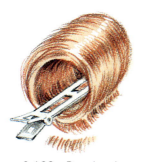

9.122—Barrel curl.

136  STANDARD TEXTBOOK OF COSMETOLOGY

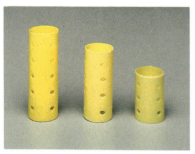

9.123—Rollers of similar width and various lengths.

Volume and Indentation

Volume is created by the base of the curl (the direction of the hair up from the head) and the size of roller. (Fig. 9.123)

1. For *full volume* (angle of strand), the roller sits on its base, or is overdirected. (See Figs. 9.124, 9.125)

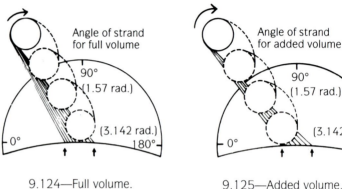

9.124—Full volume.   9.125—Added volume.

2. For *medium volume,* the roller rests ½" (1.25 cm) off the base. (It is slightly underdirected.) (See Fig. 9.126)

3. *For a small amount of lift,* the roller sits off the base. (It is underdirected.) (See Fig. 9.127)

4. To create *indentation or hollowness,* keep the hair close to the head and roll to ½" (1.25 cm) off the base. (See Fig. 9.128)

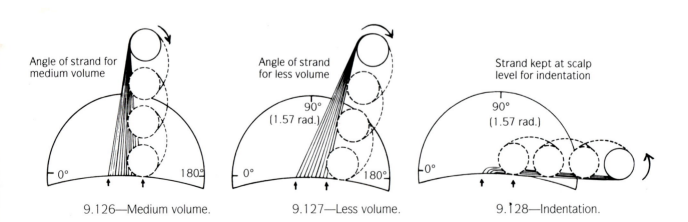

9.126—Medium volume.   9.127—Less volume.   9.128—Indentation.

5. Figs. 9.129 to 9.132 demonstrate how a finished style can be created by setting for volume and indentation.

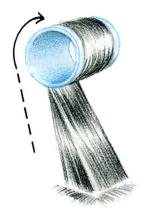

9.129a—Creates volume.

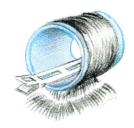

9.129b—Anchor with clip.

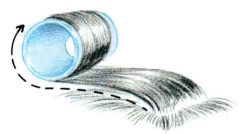

9.130a—Creates indentation or hollowness.

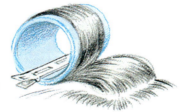

9.130b—Anchor with clip.

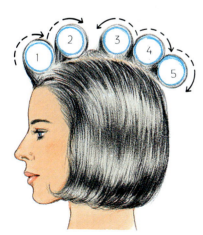

9.131—Setting pattern: 1st two rollers—volume; 3rd roller—indentation; 4th and 5th rollers—volume.

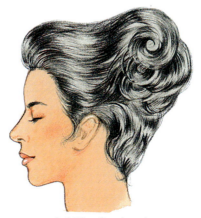

9.132—Comb-out.

Cylinder Circular Roller Action

Hair that is directed in a circular fashion is referred to by various names, such as radial motion, circular movement, curvature movement, curvature roller action, rotary motion or movement, spotmatic movement, contour movement, and so on.

The spot or area from which the hair is directed to form a circular movement is also referred to by any of the following terms: balance point, swing point, terminal point, pivot point, pendulum point, radial point, fulcrum point, radiation point, rotary point, and spotmatic point.

Roller action is created by the way the hair is molded around the roller. This roller action can be varied by using different size rollers and setting patterns. (Figs. 9.133–9.146)

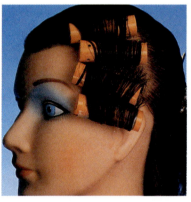
9.133—Short hair (slender rollers).

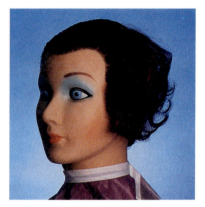
9.134—Comb-out.

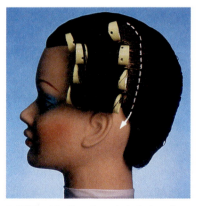
9.135—Medium length hair (medium size rollers).

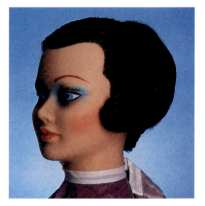
9.136—Comb-out.

CHAPTER 9 WET HAIRSTYLING ◆ 139

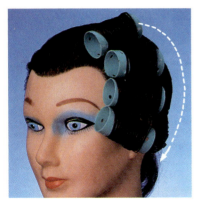

9.137—Long hair (large rollers).

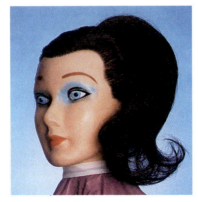

9.138—Comb-out.

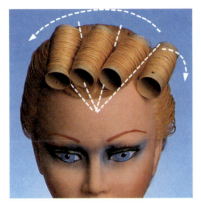

9.139—Top—cylinder rollers set in wedge-shaped partings in a circular manner.

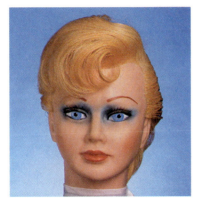

9.140—Comb-out in a forward shell effect with bangs.

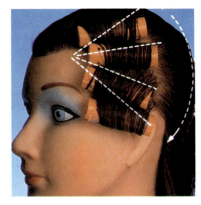

9.141—Side—cylinder rollers set in wedge-shaped partings.

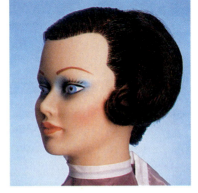

9.142—The comb-out gives a circular movement toward the face.

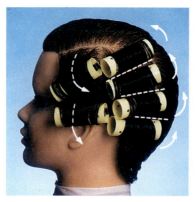

9.143—Special side effects—side roller setting with sculpture curl in front of ear.

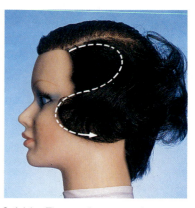

9.144—The comb-out produces an "S" wave formation effect.

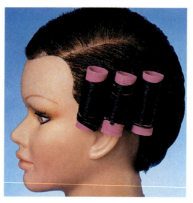

9.145—To create a ridge line and indentation (hollowness), set the hair on rollers at an angle.

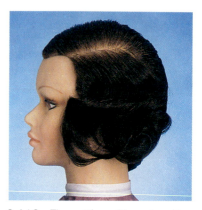

9.146—The setting will produce the waved effect in the comb-out.

Tapered Rollers

You can achieve practically the same styling results by using either cylinder or tapered rollers. However, since cylinder rollers must be placed slightly farther back from the point of distribution in a pie-shaped pattern, the movement of the hair might be weaker. The tapered roller, however, makes it possible to develop a stronger curvature movement.

Choose roller size according to the texture of your client's hair and the size of curl you desire. Fine hair requires smaller rollers; coarse hair needs larger rollers. (Figs. 9.147–9.149)

9.147—Tapered roller.

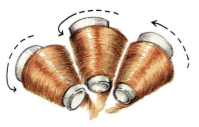
9.148—One-quarter circle setting using thinner rollers produces tighter comb-outs.

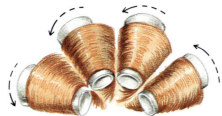
9.149—One-half circle setting using larger (thicker) rollers produces looser comb-outs.

Effect of Tapered Rollers

Tapered rollers set along the hairline produce a shell-shaped front with bangs or curled up ends. (Figs. 9.150, 9.151)

Tapered rollers set along the side of the head comb out in a forward movement. (Figs. 9.152, 9.153)

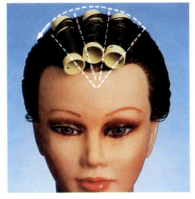
9.150—Tapered roller setting.

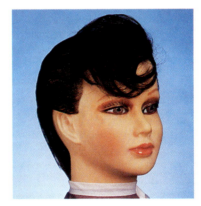
9.151—Comb-out.

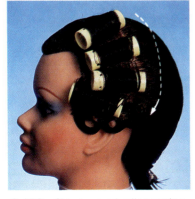
9.152—Side tapered roller setting.

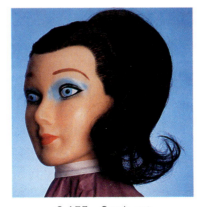
9.153—Comb-out.

Professional Prep

HOW TO WRITE A RESUME

You've passed your boards, and now you're ready for that first job. Everyone wants to see a resume, and in many cases it's your first chance to advertise your skills. The way you present it gives your future employer a clue as to how you do everything else.

Your resume should include your name, address, and phone number; your work history, including summer and part-time jobs; your educational background; and your skills and achievements. It should also include your employment objective (what job you want) and references from teachers, past or present employers, supervisors, or coworkers (not relatives or personal friends).

When organizing all this information, remember to place what is most relevant to the job you want in the most prominent position, so it will catch the employer's eye. Be sure to use active verbs to demonstrate your achievements—words like completed, created, designed, developed, produced, trained, won, etc.

Keep the information simple, clear, and positive; no one wants to wade through a lot of flowery language. Be sure to type your resume, and proofread it carefully—or have someone else proofread it, if grammar and spelling are your weaknesses.

Don't include personal information (age, marital status, parental status, race, religion, or physical characteristics), since it could work against you. (Employers are forbidden to ask about these things.)

Don't emphasize how much money you want (this will be discussed in the job interview) or what you need; instead, focus on how you can fill your employer's needs and wants.

—*From* Communication Skills for Cosmetologists *by Kathleen Ann Bergant*

COMB-OUT TECHNIQUES

Smooth and well-executed comb-outs result from perfect sets. To achieve success as a hairstylist, you must first master the skills of shaping and molding hair, then you must practice fast, simple, and effective methods for comb-outs.

Recommended Procedure

If you follow a definite system of combing out hairstyles, you will save time, be effective, and build an appreciative and loyal clientele. One procedure for combing out is outlined here.

1. After removing the rollers and clips, brush the hair through to integrate roller and pin curl settings, and relax the set. A cushioned paddle brush works well. Smooth and brush the hair into a semi-flat condition that permits you to position the lines for the planned hairstyle. It is essential that this procedure is correctly executed to achieve a smooth, flowing, finished coiffure.

2. After you have thoroughly brushed the hair, direct it into the general pattern desired. This can be accomplished by placing your hand on the client's head and gently pushing the hair forward in order that waves fall into the planned design. Lines of direction should be slightly overemphasized to allow for some expected relaxation during the comb-out process.

3. Back comb areas that require volume and back brush sections that need to be integrated. Accentuate and develop lines and style. Take one section at a time, placing the proper lines, ridges, volume, and indentations into the hairstyle. You can create softness and evenness of flow by blending, smoothing, and combing. Exaggerations and overemphasis should be eliminated. Finished patterns should reveal rhythm, balance, and smoothness of line.

4. Final touches make hairstyles look professional; *take your time*. After completing the comb-out, you can use the tail of a comb to lift areas where the shape and form are not precise. Every touch during the final stage must be very lightly performed. When the finishing touches have been completed, check the entire set for structural balance and then *lightly* spray the hair.

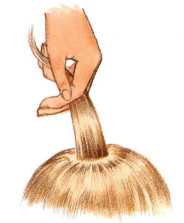

9.154—The hair properly held between the index and middle fingers.

Back-Combing and Back-Brushing Techniques

You might have to create areas of full volume in some hairstyles. Back-combing and back-brushing are the best means to achieve lift. These techniques incorporate the matting of the hair by combing or brushing it toward the scalp so that the shorter hair mats to form a cushion or base for the top or covering hair.

Back-combing is also called teasing, ratting, matting, or French lacing. It is a technique used to build a *firm* cushion on which to build full-volume curls or bouffant hairstyles.

After the basic comb-out has been directed into the desired pattern, analyze the areas that need volume.

1. Pick up a section of hair about ¾" (1.875 cm) wide and hold up firmly, away from the scalp. (Fig. 9.154)
2. Insert a fine-toothed comb into the strand about 1½" (3.75 cm) from its base, press to the scalp, and remove.
3. Repeat step 2 by inserting the comb into the strand a little farther away from the scalp and pressing firmly toward the scalp. Repeat this step as many times as necessary, using very small strokes until the desired volume of cushioned hair has been achieved.
4. Smooth the hair ends to conceal back-combing. (Figs. 9.155–9.156)

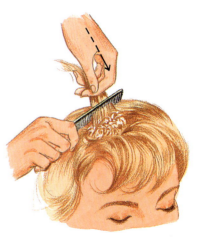

9.155—Back-combing on top of strand.

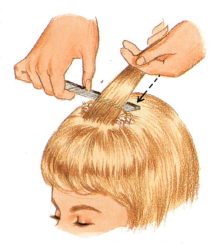

9.156—Back-combing in back of strand.

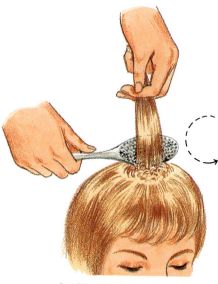

Back-brushing is also called ruffing. It is a technique used to build a *soft* cushion, or to mesh two or more curl patterns together for a uniform and smooth comb-out.

1. Pick up and hold a strand straight out from the scalp.
2. With a slight amount of slack in the strand, place a narrow brush near the base of the strand. Push and roll the inner edge of the brush with the wrist until it touches the scalp. For interlocking to occur, the brush must be rolled. Then remove the brush from the hair with a turn of the wrist, peeling back a layer of hair. The shorter ends of tapered hair are interlocked to form a cushion at the scalp.
3. Repeat this procedure by moving the brush about ½" (1.25 cm) farther away from the scalp with each stroke until the desired volume has been achieved. (Fig. 9.157)

9.157—Back-brushing.

BRAIDING

You will be asked to braid, plait, or cornrow the hair of children and adults alike. These styles must be done with a *firm* hand using even tension to all strands. It is advisable to braid on damp hair because some degree of stretch will assist in producing a long-lasting and neat style.

French Braiding

There are two different types of French braids: the *invisible braid* or regular braid and the *visible braid* or inverted braid.

Invisible braiding is performed by overlapping the strands on top.

1. Section the hair into two parts with a center part. (See Fig. 9.158)
2. Clamp one side and divide the other side into three strands. (See Fig. 9.159)

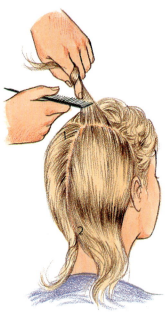

9.158—Section hair.

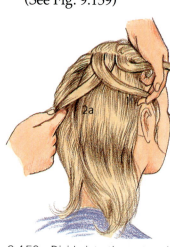

9.159—Divide into three strands.

3. Start the braid by taking strand 1 (from the left) and crossing it *over* strand 2 (center strand) (strand 1 becomes the center strand). (See Fig. 9.160)
4. Take strand 3 (from the right) and cross it *over* the center strand (it becomes the center strand). Hold the strands tightly. You have now completed the anchor point.
5. Pick up the strand on the left (original strand 2) and incorporate a small section (strand 2b), about ½" (1.25 cm) wide, from the scalp. Join the new section with the left strand and together draw them over the center strand. (See Fig. 9.161)
6. Bring original strand 1 over the center hair. Bring a strand of scalp hair from the right, about ½" (1.25 cm) wide, and place it with strand 1.
7. Continue to pick up strands and braid until all the hair in the section has been taken into the braid. (See Fig. 9.162)

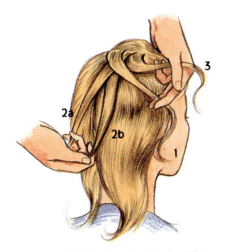

9.160—Starting the braiding.

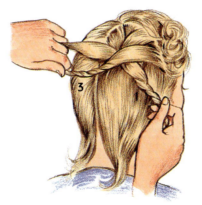

9.161—Drawing over center strand.

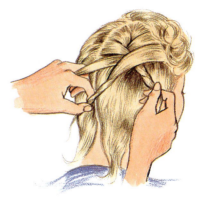

9.162—Pick up strand.

◆ **NOTE:** To keep the braid neat with all short hair ends in place, twist each strand toward the center as you put it in place.

8. Braid the other side in the same manner. (See Fig. 9.163)
9. If the hair is long you can:
   • Continue to braid through to the ends. It can then be crossed and extended up the back of the head or left to hang loose.
   • Stop the braid at the hairline and tie ribbons, allowing the ends to fall into curls.

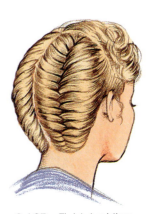

9.163—Finish braiding.

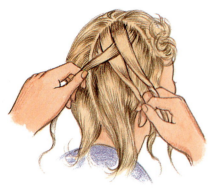

9.164—Divide into three sections and begin braiding.

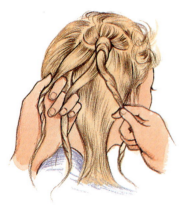

9.165—Drawing under center strand.

If the hair is not very long you can:
- Fasten the ends with a rubber band and tuck them under and pin in place with bobby pins.
- Create design lines that travel around the head from temple to temple, or form various patterns with the braids and parting lines.
- You might want to start the French braid at the nape and work toward the face. You can tuck the ends under or finish the style with curls.

Visible French braiding (inverted braid) is done by plaiting the strands under, thus making the braid visible. It is done in the same manner as the invisible braid except that strands are placed *under* the center strand.

Part and section the hair in the same manner as for regular French braid.

1. Divide the top right section evenly into three strands. Start to braid the hair strands by placing the right side strand under the center strand and the left side strand under this one. Draw strands tightly. (See Fig. 9.164)
2. Pick up ½" (1.25 cm) strand on the right side and combine with the right side strand. Place this combined strand under the center strand. Pick up ½" (1.25 cm) strand on the left side and combine with the left side strand. Place this combined strand under the center strand. (See Fig. 9.165)
3. Continue to pick up hair and braid as above. Finish braiding at nape, and hold in position with rubber bands. (See Fig. 9.166)
4. Braid left side of the head in the same manner as right side. (See Fig. 9.167)
5. The finished braids may be tucked under and held in place with hairpins or bobby pins. (See Fig. 9.168)

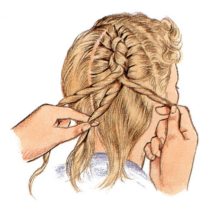

9.166—Continue braiding.

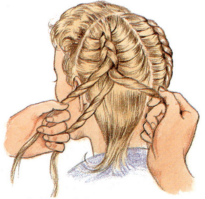

9.167—Finish braiding.

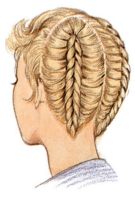

9.168—Finished look.

Cornrowing is done in the same fashion as *visible French braiding* except that the sections are very narrow and form a predetermined style. It works well with overly curly hair and is popular with both children and adults. Cornrowing should last for several weeks.

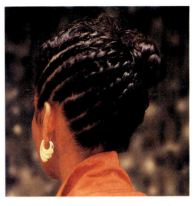

9.169—A finished cornrow style.

Preparation for Overly Curly Hair
If your client has overly curly hair, you can prepare to cornrow as follows:

1. Shampoo in the usual way.
2. Apply conditioner and distribute it well.
3. Tie a hair net over the hair to hold it flat.
4. Place your client under a hood dryer, or blow-dry the hair.
5. Follow the visible French braid procedure using narrower sections and more tension to form the cornrow braids. (Fig. 9.169)

✓ **Completed—Learning Objective No. 3**

HAIRSTYLING PROCEDURES, IMPLEMENT CARE AND USE

ARTISTRY IN HAIRSTYLING

The principles of modern hairstyling and makeup are your guides to selecting what is most appropriate in order to achieve a beautiful appearance. The best results are obtained when each client's facial features are properly analyzed for strengths and shortcomings. Your job is to accentuate a client's best features and play down features that do not add to the person's attractiveness.

You must develop the ability to analyze hairstyles for your clients. Each client deserves a hairstyle that is properly proportioned to her body type, is correctly balanced to the head and facial features, and attractively frames the face. The essentials of an artistic and suitable hairstyle are based on the following general characteristics:

1. Shape of the head: front view (face shape), profile, and back view.
2. Characteristics of features: perfect as well as imperfect features, defects, or blemishes.
3. Body structure, posture, and poise.

FACIAL TYPES
Each client's facial shape is determined by the position and prominence of the facial bones. There are seven facial shapes: oval, round, square, oblong, pear-shaped, heart-shaped, and diamond-shaped. To recognize each facial shape and to be able to give correct advice, you should be acquainted with the outstanding characteristics of each.

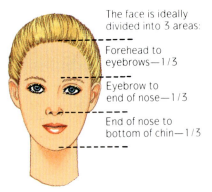

9.170—Ideal facial proportions.

The face is ideally divided into 3 areas:
Forehead to eyebrows—1/3
Eyebrow to end of nose—1/3
End of nose to bottom of chin—1/3

The face is divided into three zones: forehead to eyebrow, eyebrows to end of nose, and end of nose to bottom of chin. When creating a style for a client, you will be trying to create the illusion that each client has the ideal face shape. (Fig. 9.170)

Oval Facial Type

The oval-shaped face is generally recognized as the ideal shape. The contour and proportions of the oval face form the basis for modifying all other facial types.

Facial contour: The oval face is about 1½ times longer than its width across the brow. The forehead is slightly wider than the chin.

A person with an oval-shaped face can wear any hairstyle unless there are other considerations, such as eyeglasses, length and shape of nose, or profile. (See sections on special considerations.) (Fig. 9.171)

Round Facial Type

Facial contour: Round hairline and round chin line; wide face.

Aim: To create the illusion of length to the face.

Create a hairstyle with height by arranging the hair on top of the head. You can place some hair over the ears and cheeks, but it is also appropriate to keep the hair up on one side, leaving the ears exposed. Style the bangs to one side. (Fig. 9.172)

Square Facial Type

Facial contour: Straight hairline and square jawline; wide face.

Aims: To create the illusion of length; offset the square features.

The problems of the square facial type are similar to the round facial type. The style should lift off the forehead and come forward at the temples and jaw, creating the illusion of narrowness and softness in the face. Asymmetrical hairstyles work well. (Fig. 9.173)

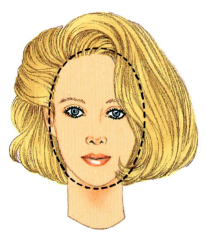

9.171—Oval face.

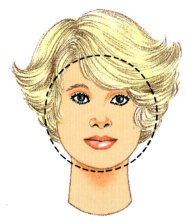

9.172—Round face.

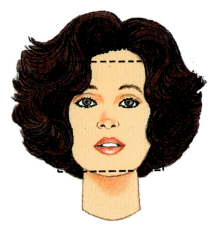

9.173—Square face.

Pear-Shaped Facial Type

Facial contour: Narrow forehead, wide jaw and chin line.

   Aim: To create the illusion of width in the forehead.

   Build a hairstyle that is fairly full and high. Cover the forehead partially with a fringe of soft hair. The hair should be worn with a semi-curl or soft wave effect cropped over the ears. This arrangement adds apparent width to the forehead. (Fig. 9.174)

Oblong Facial Type

Facial contour: Long, narrow face with hollow cheeks.

   Aim: To make the face appear shorter and wider.

   The hair should be styled fairly close to the top of the head with a fringe of curls and bangs, combined with fullness to the sides. Drawing the hair out from the cheeks creates the illusion of width. (Fig. 9.175)

Diamond Facial Type

Facial contour: Narrow forehead, extreme width through the cheekbones, and narrow chin.

   Aim: To reduce the width across the cheekbone line.

   Increasing the fullness across the jawline and forehead while keeping the hair close to the head at the cheekbone line helps create an oval appearance. Avoid hairstyles that lift away from the cheeks or move back from the hairline. (Fig. 9.176)

Heart-Shaped Facial Type

Facial contour: Wide forehead and narrow chin line.

   Aims: To decrease the width of the forehead and increase the width in the lower part of the face.

   To reduce the width of the forehead, a center part with bangs flipped up or a style slanted to one side is recommended. Add width and softness at the jawline. (Fig. 9.177)

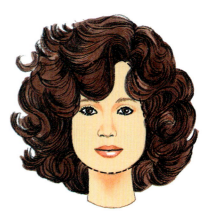

9.174—Pear-shaped face.

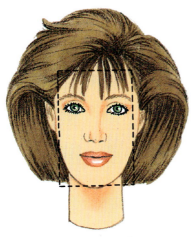

9.175—Oblong face.

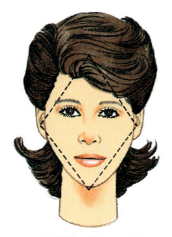

9.176—Diamond face.

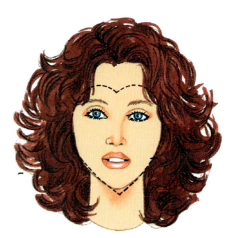

9.177—Heart-shaped face.

Profiles

Always look at your client's profile. When creating a hairstyle, the profile can be a good indicator as to the correct shape of hairstyle to choose.

Straight profile. This is considered the ideal. It is neither concave nor convex, with no unusual facial features. Usually, all hairstyles are becoming to the straight or normal profile. (Fig. 9.178)

Concave (prominent chin). The hair at the nape should be styled softly with a movement upward. Do not build hair out onto the forehead. (Fig. 9.179)

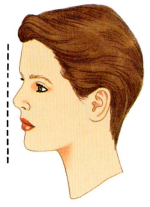 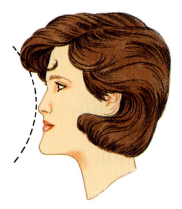

9.178—Straight profile.   9.179—Concave (prominent chin).

Convex (receding forehead, prominent nose, and receding chin). Place curls or bangs over the forehead. Keep the style close to the head at the nape. (Fig. 9.180)

Low forehead, protruding chin. Create an illusion of fullness to the forehead by building a fluffy bang with height. An upswept temple movement will add length to the face. Soft curls in the nape area soften the chin line. Do not end the style line at the nape—this draws attention to the chin line. Rather, create a line that is either higher or lower than the chin line. (Fig. 9.181)

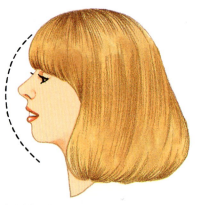 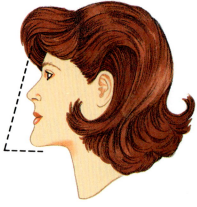

9.180—Convex (receding forehead, prominent nose, and receding chin).   9.181—Low forehead, protruding chin.

Nose Shapes

Nose shapes are closely related to profile. When studying your client's face, the nose must be considered both in profile and in full face. (Appropriate makeup for nose shapes will be found in the chapter on facial makeup.)

Turned-up nose. This type of nose is usually small and accompanied by a straight profile. The small nose is considered to be a childlike quality; therefore it is best to design a hairstyle that is not associated with children. The hair should be swept off the face creating a line from the nose to the ear. This will add length to the short nose. The top hair should move off the forehead to give the illusion of length to the nose. (Figs. 9.182, 9.183)

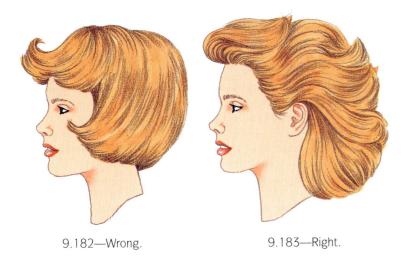

9.182—Wrong.   9.183—Right.

Prominent nose (hooked, large, or pointed). In order to draw attention away from the nose, bring the hair forward at the forehead with softness around the face. (Figs. 9.184, 9.185)

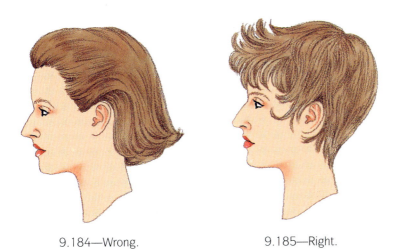

9.184—Wrong.   9.185—Right.

Crooked nose. To minimize the conspicuous crooked nose, style the hair in an off-center manner that will attract the eye away from the nose. Asymmetrical styles are best. Any well-balanced hairstyle will accentuate the fact that the face is not even. (Figs. 9.186, 9.187)

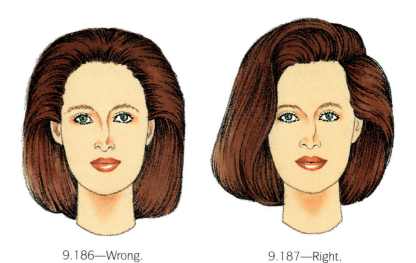

9.186—Wrong. 9.187—Right.

Wide, flat nose. A wide, flat nose tends to broaden the face. In order to minimize this effect, the hair should be drawn away from the face. In addition, a center part tends to narrow the nose, as well as draw attention away from the nose. (Figs. 9.188, 9.189)

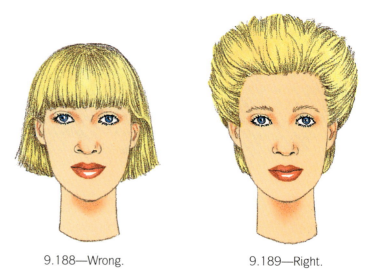

9.188—Wrong. 9.189—Right.

Eyes

The eyes are the focal point of a face. Be prepared to create hairstyles that bring out the best in a client's eyes.

Wide-set eyes are usually found on a round or square face. You can minimize the effect by lifting and fluffing the top of the hair and bang area. A side bang helps to draw attention away from the space between the eyes. (Figs. 9.190, 9.191)

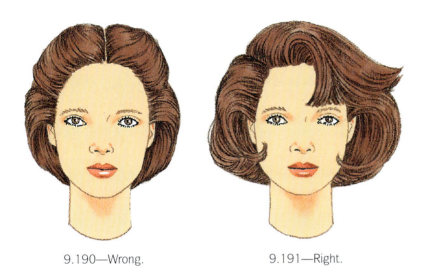

9.190—Wrong.　　　　　9.191—Right.

Close-set eyes are usually found on long, narrow faces. Try to open the face with the illusion of more space between the eyes. Style the hair fairly high with a side movement. The hair ends should turn outward and up. (Figs. 9.192, 9.193)

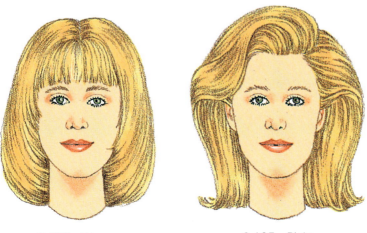

9.192—Wrong.　　　　　9.193—Right.

Head Shapes

The shape of your client's head is just as individual as other physical features. As with the face, the oval is considered the ideal shape. Your goal when designing hairstyles should be to give them the illusion of an oval. As you evaluate your client's head shape, mentally impose an oval picture over it. Where there is flatness, plan to build volume. (Figs. 9.194–9.199)

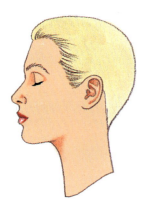

9.194—The perfect oval.

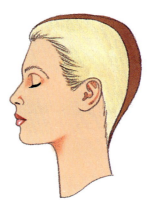

9.195—Narrow head—flat back.

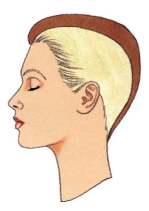

9.196—Flat crown.

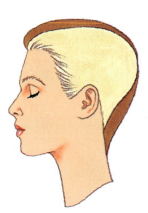

9.197—Pointed head, hollow nape.

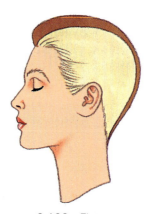

9.198—Flat top.

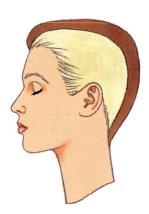

9.199—Small head.

Special Considerations

Very few, if any, of your clients will have a perfect set of features. Your goal is to analyze their features and accentuate the best ones. In addition you will need to consider the particular features of various ethnic groups.

Plump with short neck

Aim: To create the illusion of length.

Corrective hairstyle: Sweep the hair up to give length to the neck. Build height on top. Avoid hairstyles that give fullness to the back of the neck and hairstyles with horizontal lines. (Fig. 9.200)

Long, thin neck

Aim: To minimize the appearance of the long neck.

Corrective hairstyle: Cover the neck with soft waves. Avoid short or sculptured necklines. Keep the hair long and full at the nape. (Fig. 9.201)

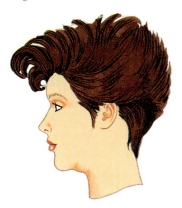
9.200—Plump with short neck.

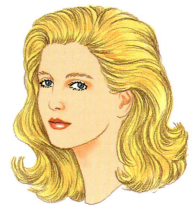
9.201—Long, thin neck.

Thin features

Aim: To give width to the face and neck.

Corrective hairstyle: Lift sides up and away from the hairline, but keep the style soft and loose. The nape hair should be long and full to fill in at the neck. (Fig. 9.202)

Uneven features

Aim: To minimize imperfect features.

Corrective hairstyle: Any style that draws attention away from the imperfect features. If a face is smaller on one side than on the other, an asymmetrical style may balance it. (Fig. 9.203)

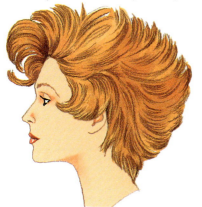
9.202—Thin features.

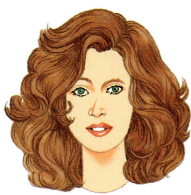
9.203—Uneven features.

Multi-cultural clients

Follow styling rules that relate to the particular face shape. If the hair has been straightened, set it on large rollers. If not, press it thermally with a large barrel iron (see chapter on thermal hairstyling). Either method will allow you to gain more control in order to style the hair according to hair art principles. (Fig. 9.204) Keep in mind that oriental hair is usually strong and may require more precise handling. (Fig. 9.205)

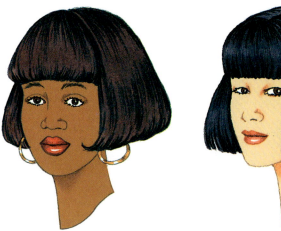
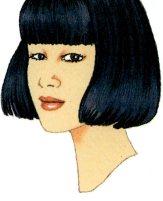

9.204—Black client.   9.205—Oriental client.

STYLING FOR PEOPLE WHO WEAR GLASSES

People who wear glasses have special issues regarding their hairstyling and makeup habits. A combination of a becoming hairstyle, the proper makeup, and the correct glasses will help to accentuate the wearer's best features.

The following are a number of basic good grooming rules that should be followed by all people who wear glasses:

1. Glass frames should be up-to-date, with large lenses for good vision.
2. Never wear gaudy, over-jewelled, or tricky frames.
3. Do not wear strip false eyelashes. They are too long and function like windshield wipers with every eye movement.
4. Do not use heavy eye makeup. It does not require heavy makeup to bring out the color and the best features of your eyes.
5. Hairstyles should fall naturally around the face, to make putting on and taking off glasses easy.
6. Over-styled hair with many tight curls is impractical for people with glasses.

The following are some of the "do's" for people who wear glasses:

The Round, Oval, or Square Face

Glasses. A person with big eyes should wear slender frames with large visual lenses to show off eyes and good eye makeup. The color of frames should be selected carefully to match hair color.

Hairstyle. A bouffant hairstyle in natural balance; a simple, uncluttered, casual style is best.

Bangs. A slashed bang freely touching the eyebrows is best.

Jewelry. If earrings are worn, they should be long and dangling. (Figs. 9.206, 9.207)

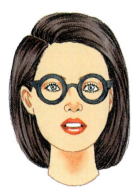
9.206—Wrong.

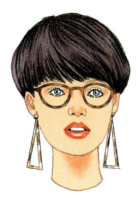
9.207—Right.

The Heart-Shaped or Diamond-Shaped Face

Glasses. The frames should be slender, of medium thickness, follow the eyebrows, and rest gently against the face.

Makeup. Wear light makeup shades and delicate eye makeup.

Hairstyle. A full pageboy style; or increase the width in the lower part of the face.

Bangs. Open bangs harmonize and balance with the lower part of the face. (Figs. 9.208, 9.209)

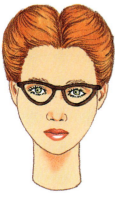
9.208—Wrong.

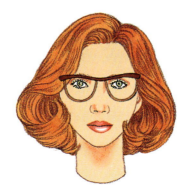
9.209—Right.

The Small, Narrow, or Oval Face

Glasses. Select large, up-to-date frames that are not too gaudy.

Makeup. Wear only natural tones of makeup. The eyes are seen and magnified through the glasses. Proper eye makeup emphasizes beautiful, sparkling eyes.

Hairstyle. Since the face is delicate in proportion, it is important that the hairstyle have width and height. The hairstyle should be short, with deep wave shapings on the sides, leaving freedom for control of glasses.

Bangs. A side wave bang caressing one eyebrow can complement the eyes. (Figs. 9.210, 9.211)

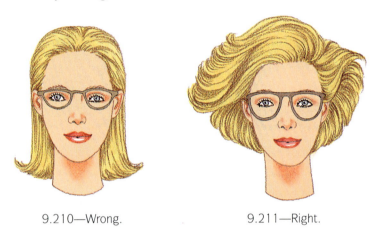

9.210—Wrong.   9.211—Right.

The Pear-Shaped Face

Glasses. Wear large, oval-shaped frames to let the glasses reveal eyes wearing appropriate makeup.

Hairstyle. This facial contour requires emphasis on length; therefore, wear the hair up and off the face, high in the front and crown. Soft bouffant styling around the face, with softness brushed forward on the cheeks, reduces width and adds beauty.

Bangs. A side wave bang over one eye will add expression and interest. (Figs. 9.212, 9.213)

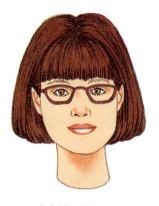 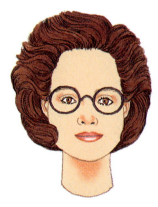

9.212—Wrong.   9.213—Right.

HAIR PARTINGS

Hair partings can be the focal point of a hairstyle. Because the eye is drawn to a part you must be careful how you use it. It must always be neat, without hairs straggling from one side or another, and it must be straight and directed positively. It is usually best to use a natural part if at all possible; however, you may want to create a parting according to your client's head shape, facial features, or desired hairstyle. It is often difficult to create a lasting hairstyle when working against the natural crown parting. You might be able to incorporate the natural parting into the finished style.

The following are suggestions for suitable hair partings for various facial types.

Partings for Bangs

1. *Rectangular* or *triangular partings* are most commonly used for children's bangs. The triangular parting distributes more hair to the temple area, which is often sparse in children.

2. *Diagonal part* used to give height to a round or square face. It also gives width to a long, thin face. (Fig. 9.214)

3. *Curved rectangular part* used for receding hairline or high forehead. (Fig. 9.215)

4. *Center part* for popular children's hairstyle with bangs. (Fig. 9.216)

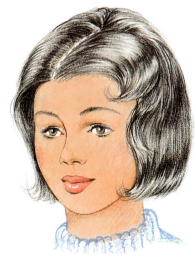
9.214—Diagonal part.

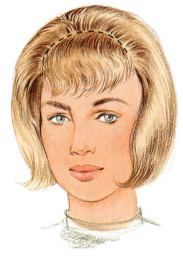
9.215—Curved rectangular part.

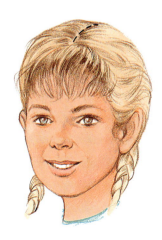
9.216—Center part for child.

Style Parts

1. *Concealed part,* used for height and a one-sided style effect. (Fig. 9.217)
2. *Side parts* are used for styles that are directed to one side. You might want to use a high side parting if your client has a wide forehead and a low side parting or diagonal parting for a triangular, round, or square-shaped face. (Fig. 9.218)
3. *Center partings* are classical. They are usually used for an oval face, but give an oval illusion to wide, round, and heart-shaped faces. (Fig. 9.219)
4. Partings can be used on other parts of the head to create avant-garde looks. *Diagonal back parting* (Fig. 9.220) and *natural crown partings* (Figs. 9.221, 9.222) used for clients with thin, long necks to create the illusion of width to the back of the head.

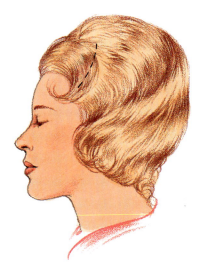

9.217—Concealed part.

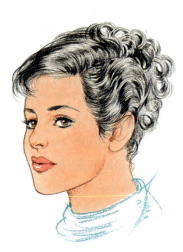

9.218—Side part.

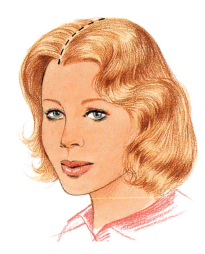

9.219—Center parting.

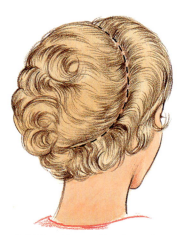

9.220—Diagonal back parting.

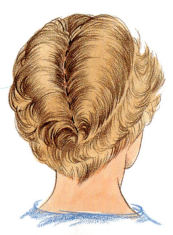

9.221—Natural crown parting—full length of head.

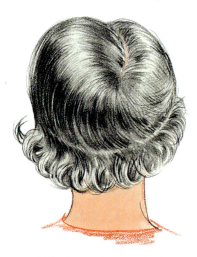

9.222—Natural crown parting—mid-way.

CHAPTER 9   WET HAIRSTYLING   ◆   161

Learning to employ skills that produce predictable results will bring you success as a professional hairstylist. You can use the art and technique of shaping, molding, setting, and brushing and combing to create any hairstyle that comes into fashion. You will easily build an appreciative and loyal clientele if you are sensitive to and make suitable compensations for imperfections in your client's features. ✔

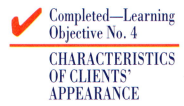

Completed—Learning Objective No. 4

CHARACTERISTICS OF CLIENTS' APPEARANCE

REVIEW QUESTIONS

WET HAIRSTYLING

1. What is hairstyling? *page 112*
2. List the basic elements of art that you use to style hair. *page 112*
3. What does a hairstyle consist of? *page 112*
4. List the implements employed in hairstyling. *page 112*
5. List the principal parts of a pin curl. *page 114*
6. What is a shaping for pin curl placement and how is it classified? *page 116*
7. List the most commonly used bases of a pin curl. *page 118–119*
8. List the bases of a roller curl. *page 132*
9. What ability must you develop to analyze your client? *page 147*

Answers to Review Questions

Chapter 1
YOUR PROFESSIONAL IMAGE
(Answers to Questions on Page 22)

1. rest, exercise, relaxation, nutrition, personal hygiene, and personal grooming

2. posture, walk, and movements

3. Personality is the outward reflection of inner feelings, thoughts, attitudes, and values.

4. listening skills, voice, speech, manner of speaking, and conversational skills

5. the psychology of getting along well with others

6. A professional attitude is expressed by self-esteem, confidence in one's profession, and respect for others.

7. the study of standards of conduct and moral judgment

Chapter 2
BACTERIOLOGY
(Answers to Questions on Page 30)

1. Bacteriology is necessary to protect individual and public health.

2. Bacteriology is the science that deals with the study of microorganisms called bacteria.

3. Bacteria are minute, one-celled vegetable microorganisms found nearly everywhere.

4. Bacteria can exist almost anywhere, for example, on the skin, in water, air, decayed matter, secretions of body openings, on clothing, and beneath the nails.

5. a) nonpathogenic bacteria—helpful, harmless, perform useful functions such as decomposing refuse b) pathogenic bacteria—harmful, produce disease when they invade plant or animal tissue

6. Parasites are harmful pathogenic bacteria that require living matter for their growth. Saprophytes are helpful nonpathogenic bacteria that live on dead matter and do not produce disease.

7. a) Cocci are round-shaped organisms that appear singly. b) Bacilli are rod-shaped organisms. They are the most common bacteria and produce diseases. c) Spirilla are curved or corkscrew-shaped organisms.

8. a) Staphylococci are pus-forming organisms that grow in bunches or clusters. They cause abscesses, pustules, and boils. b) Streptococci are pus-forming organisms that grow in chains. They cause infections such as strep throat. c) Diplococci grow in pairs and cause pneumonia.

9. Bacteria grow and reproduce under favorable conditions with sufficient food. When they reach their largest size, they divide into two new cells by a process called mitosis.

10. During the active or vegetative stage, bacteria grow and reproduce. During the inactive, spore-forming stage, no growth or reproduction occurs.

11. by hairlike projections called flagella or cilia

12. a) A local infection is indicated by a boil or pimple that contains pus. b) A general infection results when the bloodstream carries the bacteria to all parts of the body, as in syphilis.

13. one that can be spread from one person to another by contact

14. Infections can be prevented and controlled through personal hygiene and public sanitation.

15. a) Plant parasites can produce contagious diseases, such as ringworm and favus (a skin disease of the scalp). b) Animal parasites can produce contagious diseases, such as scabies and pediculosis (infection of the scalp by lice).

16. Immunity is the ability of the body to destroy bacteria that have gained entrance and thus to resist infection. The two types are natural immunity and acquired immunity.

17. Bacteria can be destroyed by disinfectants and by intense heat.

Chapter 3
DECONTAMINATION AND INFECTION CONTROL
(Answers to Questions on Page 42)

1. removing pathogens and other substances from tools or surfaces

2. Sterilization completely destroys all living organisms on a surface, even bacterial spores, the most resistant form of life on Earth.

3. Sanitation means to significantly reduce the number of pathogens fround on a surface. Salon tools and other surfaces are sanitized by cleaning with soaps or detergents.

4. Antiseptics can kill bacteria or slow their growth. Antiseptics are weaker than disinfectants and are safe

for application to skin. Disinfectants kill microbes on contaminated tools and other nonliving surfaces. Disinfectants are not for use on human skin, hair, or nails.

5. All disinfectants must be approved by the EPA and each individual state. The disinfectant's label must also have an EPA registration number.
6. MSDSs (Material Safety Data Sheets) provide all pertinent information on products, ranging from content and associated hazards, to combustion levels and storage requirements. They are available from a product's distributor.
7. They must be bactericides to kill harmful bacteria and fungicides to destroy fungus.
8. a) quaternary ammonium compounds (quats) b) phenolic disinfectants (phenols) c) alcohol d) bleach (sodium hypochlorite)
9. Bar soap can actually grow bacteria. It is much more sanitary to provide pump-type liquid, antiseptic soaps.
10. Formaldehyde, the gas released from formalin tablets or liquids, is a suspected human cancer-causing agent. It is poisonous to inhale and is extremely irritating to the eyes, nose, throat, and lungs.
11. Universal sanitation is the use of gloves and safety glasses, disinfectants and detergents in conjunction with personal hygiene and salon cleanliness.

Chapter 4
PROPERTIES OF THE SCALP AND HAIR
(Answers to Questions on Page 66)

1. The chief purposes of hair are adornment and protection of the head from heat, cold, and injury.
2. Hair is an appendage of the skin, a slender, threadlike outgrowth of the skin and scalp.
3. Hair is composed chiefly of the protein keratin, which is found in all horny growths, including the nails and skin.
4. the hair root and the hair shaft
5. The rate of growth of human hair differs on specific parts of the body, between sexes, among races, and with age. Hair growth is also influenced by seasons of the year, nutrition, health, and hormones.
6. Factors such as sex, age, type of hair, heredity, and health have a bearing on the duration of hair life. The area of an average head is about 120 square inches. There is an average of 1,000 hairs to a square inch.
7. How light or dark it is depends on the number of grains of pigment in each strand.
8. cleanliness and stimulation

Chapter 5
DRAPING
(Answers to Questions on Page 71)

1. the comfort and protection of the client
2. Draping is the means of protecting clients' skin and clothing with the use of neck strips, towels, and capes.
3. to protect skin and clothing from water, chemicals, and bacteria
4. It is used for sanitary reasons to prevent the cape from coming into direct contact with the client's skin.
5. a) prepare materials b) sanitize hands c) ask the client to remove all neck and hair jewelry and remove objects from the client's hair d) turn collar to the inside
6. For wet services, use a towel over and under the cape. For dry services, use neck strip only. For chemical services, use a towel under and above the cape.

Chapter 6
SHAMPOOING, RINSING, AND CONDITIONING
(Answers to Questions on Page 82)

1. It lets your client know that you can perform all hair services with professional competency and concern.
2. to cleanse the hair and scalp and as a preliminary step for other hair services
3. Hair should be shampooed as often as necessary to remove the accumulation of oil and perspiration, which can offer a breeding place for disease-producing bacteria.
4. Select the shampoo according to the condition of the hair.
5. hard and soft
6. It stimulates blood circulation to the scalp; helps remove dust, dirt, and hair spray; and gives hair added sheen.
7. before giving a chemical service or if scalp is irritated
8. potential hydrogen
9. The amount of hydrogen in a solution is measured on a pH scale ranging from 0 to 14; the more hydrogen present, the more alkaline the shampoo (7 to 14); the less hydrogen, the lower the pH (0 to 6.9).
10. The lower pH or acid balance prevents excessive dryness and hair damage. The higher pH or alkaline balance can leave the hair dry and brittle.
11. It is a mixture of water with a mild acid, coloring agent, or ingredients designed to serve a particular purpose.
12. It removes soap scum from the hair and restores the hair's pH balance.
13. a cream rinse

14. an acid-balanced rinse
15. by closing the cuticle and trapping color molecules
16. It is formulated to control minor dandruff conditions.
17. to highlight or add temporary color to the hair

Chapter 7
HAIRCUTTING
(Answers to Questions on Page 100)

1. Haircutting serves as a foundation for attractive hairstyles and for other services.
2. a) head shape b) facial contour c) neckline d) hair texture
3. haircutting scissors, thinning shears, straight razors with safety guards, hair clippers, combs, and clippies
4. sectioning the hair properly
5. to remove excess bulk without shortening length
6. a) fine hair—½" to 1" b) medium hair—1" to 1½" c) coarse hair—1½" to 2"
7. nape of the neck (ear to ear), side of the head (above ears), around the facial hairline, in the hair part, and near the ends of a hair strand
8. Slithering is the process of thinning hair with scissors.
9. A guideline establishes the line to be followed in shaping the balance of the head and helps to establish the general shaping pattern.
10. Shingling is cutting the hair close to the nape and gradually longer toward the crown, without showing a definite line.
11. Clippers are used to "clean" the neckline.
12. to prevent dulling the razor and to avoid pulling the hair
13. Tapering is shortening the hair in a graduated effect.
14. It should be cut dry.

Chapter 8
FINGER WAVING
(Answers to Questions on Page 109)

1. to learn the technique of moving and directing hair
2. Waving lotion makes the hair more pliable and keeps it in place during the procedure.
3. horizontal finger waving, vertical finger waving, and shadow wave
4. a) Wash hands and have available sanitized implements and supplies. b) Avoid the use of an excessive amount of waving lotion. c) Mold the waves in the direction of the natural growth. d) Protect client's forehead and ears from intense heat while under dryer with cotton, gauze, or paper protectors. e) Thoroughly dry the hair before combing it out.

Chapter 9
WET HAIRSTYLING
(Answers to Questions on Page 161)

1. Hairstyling is the process of creating wearable art.
2. weight and balance, form, rhythm, shape, composition, contrast, elevation, texture, structure, and the use of space
3. shaping or molding to create interesting patterns
4. hairpins, bobby pins, rollers and roller pins, duckbill clamps, clippies, combs, and brushes
5. The principal parts of a pin curl are the base, stem, and circle.
6. A shaping is a section of hair that is molded into a design to serve as a base for a curl or wave pattern. It is classified as forward and reverse; diagonal, vertical, or horizontal; oblong or circular.
7. rectangular, triangular, arc, and square
8. The bases of a roller curl are full volume, medium volume, and indentation.
9. the ability to analyze hairstyles for your clients according to shape of the head, characteristics of features and body structure, and facial shapes

Chapter 10
THERMAL HAIRSTYLING
(Answers to Questions on Page 186)

1. the art of waving and curling straight or pressed hair
2. a) conventional b) electric self-heated c) electric self-heated, vaporizing
3. Place a comb between iron and scalp.
4. drying and styling damp hair in one operation
5. dryer, brushes, and combs
6. styling lotion, hair conditioner, and hair spray

Chapter 11
PERMANENT WAVING
(Answers to Questions on Page 224)

1. It provides a long-lasting style; makes home styling easy; adds volume and fullness to fine hair; and gives greater control over coarse, wiry, and hard-to-manage hair.
2. wrapping hair from scalp to ends
3. wrapping hair from ends toward scalp
4. A cold wave is a perm that does not require heat.
5. a) A waving lotion softens or breaks the internal structure of the hair. b) A neutralizer rehardens or rebonds the internal structure of the hair.
6. a mild perm with pH levels ranging from 4.5 to 7.9, which penetrates the hair more slowly and uses heat to shorten the processing time

7. a process incorporated into many waving lotions to ensure optimum curl development within a fixed time, without risk of overprocessing or damaging the hair

8. a strong perm with pH levels ranging from 8.2 to 9.6, which processes at room temperature within 5 to 20 minutes, producing a strong curl

9. a) ammonium thioglycolate b) glyceryl monothioglycolate

10. exothermic

11. hydrogen peroxide, at an acidic pH

12. physical action and chemical action

13. a) cuticle—outer covering protecting the hair b) cortex—where physical and chemical action takes place; gives hair flexibility, elasticity, strength, resilience, and color c) medulla—innermost section, function unknown

14. keratin

15. disulfide bonds

16. Evaluate and analyze client's hair, and consult with client about expectations (tight or loose curl).

17. to determine if it is safe to perm and what products and technique to use

18. It is the hair's capacity to absorb liquids.

19. lotion specifically designed to even out the porosity so that even curl patterns result

20. Hair texture is the thickness or thinness (in diameter) of each individual strand.

21. a) texture b) porosity

22. It is the ability of hair to stretch and contract.

23. It refers to the number of hairs per square inch.

24. the size of the rod

25. a) concave b) straight

26. a) amount of curl desired b) physical characteristics of the hair

27. Sectioning and blocking makes work easier because it creates an overall pattern for rod placement.

28. a) The average parting should match the diameter of the rod. b) The length of blocking should be the same or a little shorter than the length of the rod.

29. It should be wrapped smoothly and neatly without stretching.

30. End wraps ensure smooth, even wrapping and minimize the danger of breakage.

31. a) double end paper wrap b) single end paper wrap c) book end wrap

32. It is a test to determine optimum curl development. Unwind the rod and check for the "S" pattern foundation.

Chapter 12
HAIRCOLORING
(Answers to Questions on Page 318)

1. Primary colors are basic or true colors that are not created by combining other colors. The three primary colors are yellow, red, and blue. Secondary colors are created by mixing equal amounts of two primary colors. Tertiary colors are created by mixing equal amounts of one primary color with one of its adjacent secondary colors.

2. The classifications of haircolor are: temporary, semi-permanent, and permanent. Temporary color can only deposit pigment, it cannot lighten. Semi-permanent color has a mild penetrating action that results in a gentle addition of color in the cortex as well as some coating of the cuticle, but does not change the basic structure of the hair. Permanent haircolor penetrates the cuticle and deposits molecules into the cortex. These colors can both lift and deposit.

3. Always record the consultation on a client record card. Consider what colors will suit the client's skin tone. Also consider the client's personality and lifestyle. Advise the client on the benefits of using a good quality shampoo and conditioner. For a strand test: mix ½ tsp. of color with peroxide. Apply mixture to a ½" section. Process. Rinse strand, shampoo, towel dry, and examine results. Adjust formula, timing, or preconditioning necessary and proceed with tinting on entire head. If results are unsatisfactory, adjust the formula and repeat process on a new test strand.

4. Apply color with applicator bottle. Apply rinse through entire hair shaft and comb through. Blend the color with a comb, applying more color as necessary.

5. The color is self-penetrating. The color is applied the same way each time. Retouching is not necessary. Color does not rub off on pillow or clothing. Hair returns to its natural color after 4 to 6 shampoos.

6. Section hair. Prepare tint. Begin where color change will be greatest. Part off ¼" subsection. Apply tint to hair ½" from scalp up to, but not through, the porous ends. Process according to strand test results. Check for color development by removing color from strand. Apply tint mixture to hair at scalp. Blend tint to hair ends. Massage color to lather and rinse thoroughly. Remove stains. Shampoo. Apply an acid or finishing rinse.

7. Client is consulted. Hair is analyzed and conditioned. Tint is applied to new growth only. Diluted color formula is applied to hair ends. Diluted tint mixture is applied to entire head if ends have faded.

8. Give a patch test 24 to 48 hours prior to any application of aniline derivative. Apply tint only if patch test is

negative. Do not apply tint if abrasions are present. Do not apply tint if metallic or compound dye is present. Do not brush hair prior to applying color. Always read and follow manufacturer's directions. Use sanitized applicator bottles, brushes, combs, and towels. Protect client's clothing by proper draping. Perform a strand test for color, breakage, and/or discoloration. Use an applicator bottle or bowl (glass or plastic) for mixing the tint. Do not mix tint before you are ready to use it; discard leftover tint. Wear gloves to protect your hands. Do not permit the color to come in contact with the client's eyes. Do not overlap during a tint retouch. Do not use water that is too hot; use lukewarm water for removing color. Use a mild shampoo. If an alkaline or harsh shampoo is used it will strip the color. Always wash hands before and after serving a client.

9. Hydrogen peroxide serves as an oxidizing agent that causes oxygen to combine with another substance, such as melanin. As the oxygen and melanin combine, the peroxide solution begins to diffuse and lighten the melanin within the hair shaft. This new smaller structure and spread-out distribution of the diffused melanin gives the hair its light appearance.

10. a) as a color treatment, to lighten the hair to the final shade desired b) as a preliminary treatment, to prepare the hair for the application of a toner or tint

11. Oil bleaches are used for lightening the entire head. Cream lighteners are popular for all types of lightening services. Powder lighteners are generally used for special effects lightening.

12. cap, foil, and freehand techniques

13. Incorporate reconditioning. Ensure that the client uses high-quality products at home. Precondition hair that is damaged. Use a penetrating conditioner. Complete each chemical service by normalizing the pH with a finishing rinse. Postpone any further chemical service until the hair is reconditioned. Schedule the client for between-service conditioning.

Chapter 13
CHEMICAL HAIR RELAXING AND SOFT CURL PERMANENT
(Answers to Questions on Page 338)

1. chemical hair relaxer, neutralizer, and a petroleum cream
2. a) sodium hydroxide b) ammonium thioglycolate
3. a) processing b) neutralizing c) conditioning
4. Follow the manufacturer's instructions.
5. a chemical blow out
6. a) scalp examination b) hair analysis c) strand test
7. soft curl permanent waving
8. a soft curl permanent
9. reconditioning treatments

Chapter 14
THERMAL HAIR STRAIGHTENING (HAIR PRESSING)
(Answers to Questions on Page 349)

1. thermal hair straightening
2. temporarily straightens overly curly or unruly hair
3. soft press, medium press, and hard press
4. scalp abrasion, contagious scalp condition, scalp injury, or chemically treated hair
5. Apply 1% gentian violet jelly.
6. Test on white cloth or white paper.
7. lightened, tinted, or gray hair

Chapter 15
THE ARTISTRY OF ARTIFICIAL HAIR
(Answers to Questions on Page 368)

1. personal choice, medical reasons, fashion, and practicality
2. human hair, synthetic hair, and animal hair
3. It makes hair look longer.
4. to give a professional result when shaping, setting, and styling
5. every 2 to 4 weeks
6. on a wig block
7. Color rinses can only darken the hair.

Chapter 16
MANICURING AND PEDICURING
(Answers to Questions on Page 400)

1. The word manicure is derived from the Latin *manus* (hand) and *cura* (care), which means the care of the hands and nails.
2. a) square b) round c) oval d) pointed
3. orangewood sticks, nail file, cuticle pusher, cuticle nipper or scissors, nail brush, and emery boards
4. from corner to center
5. It keeps the hands flexible, well-groomed, and smooth.
6. electric, oil, men's, and booth manicure
7. nail wraps, sculptured nails, nail tipping, dipping, press-on, and acrylic overlays
8. Pedicuring is the care of the feet, toes, and toenails. It has become an important client service because of the shoe styles that expose various parts of the heel and toes. Foot care not only improves personal appearance, it also adds to the comfort of the feet.

Chapter 17
THE NAIL AND ITS DISORDERS
(Answers to Questions on Page 410)

1. The normal, healthy nail is firm and flexible and appears to be slightly pink in color.
2. Onyx is the technical term for the nail.
3. The nail is composed mainly of keratin, a protein substance that forms the base of all horny tissue.
4. The nail consists of three parts: nail body, nail root, and free edge.
5. cuticle, eponychium, hyponychium, perionychium, nail walls, nail grooves, and mantle
6. The matrix is the part of the nail bed that extends beneath the nail root and contains nerves, lymph, and blood vessels to nourish the nail.
7. Any nail disease that shows signs of infection or inflammation (redness, pain, swelling, or pus) must not be treated in a beauty salon.

Chapter 18
THEORY OF MASSAGE
(Answers to Questions on Page 418)

1. Massage is used to exercise facial muscles, maintain muscle tone, and stimulate circulation.
2. Massage involves the application of external manipulations to the head and body.
3. The origin of a muscle is the fixed attachment of one end of that muscle to a bone or tissue.
4. The insertion is the attachment of the opposite end of the muscle to another muscle or to a movable bone or joint.
5. Direction of movement is generally from the insertion of a muscle toward its origin.
6. a) The skin and all its structures are nourished. b) The skin is rendered soft and pliable. c) The circulation of the blood is increased. d) The activity of the skin glands is stimulated. e) The muscle fiber is stimulated and strengthened. f) The nerves are smoothed and rested. g) Pain is sometimes relieved.
7. a) effleurage b) petrissage c) friction d) percussion or tapotement e) vibration

Chapter 19
FACIALS
(Answers to Questions on Page 438)

1. It is a restful, stimulating experience resulting in a noticeable improvement in skin tone, texture, and appearance.
2. to determine products to use, areas that need special attention, amount of pressure for massage, if lubricating oil or cream is needed around the eyes, and equipment to use
3. For sanitary reasons you should use a spatula to remove products from their containers.
4. Dry skin is the result of an insufficient flow of sebum from the sebaceous glands.
5. Another name for blackheads is comedones.
6. Oily skin and/or blackheads are caused by a hardened mass of sebum formed in the ducts of the sebaceous glands.
7. Milia or whiteheads is a common skin disorder, caused by the formation of sebaceous matter within or under the skin.
8. Acne is a disorder of the sebaceous glands; therefore it requires medical direction.
9. Mask facials are recommended for dry skin.
10. Pack facials are recommended for normal and oily skin.
11. A hot oil mask facial is recommended for dry, scaly skin, or skin that is inclined to wrinkle.

Chapter 20
FACIAL MAKEUP
(Answers to Questions on Page 472)

1. The main objective of a makeup application is to emphasize the client's most attractive facial features and to minimize less attractive features.
2. When applying makeup, you must take into consideration the structure of a client's face; the color of the eyes, skin, and hair; how the client wants to look; and the results you can achieve.
3. a) oval b) round c) square d) pear e) heart f) diamond g) oblong
4. Foundation provides a base for color harmony; evens out the skin color; conceals minor imperfections; and protects the skin from soil, wind, and weather.
5. Skin tones, or pigments, determine the selection of foundation color.
6. a) liquid b) cream c) dry (compact) d) brush-on powdered (loose)
7. only if it belongs to the client
8. to enhance natural lashes and make them appear thicker and longer
9. Corrective makeup is used to minimize unattractive features and accent good features.
10. a) strip eyelashes b) semi-permanent individual eyelashes (eye tabbing)

Chapter 21
THE SKIN AND ITS DISORDERS
(Answers to Questions on Page 490)

1. The skin is the largest and one of the most important organs of the body.

2. Healthy skin is slightly moist, soft, and flexible; possesses a slightly acid reaction; and is free from any disease or disorder.
3. a) epidermis b) dermis.
4. Blood and lymph supply nourishment to the skin.
5. The color of the skin, whether fair, medium, or dark, depends, in part, on the blood supply to the skin and primarily on melanin, the coloring matter that is deposited in the stratum germinativum and the papillary layers of the dermis.
6. The skin contains two types of duct glands that extract materials from the blood to form new substances: the sudoriferous, or sweat glands, and the sebaceous, or oil glands.
7. a) protection b) sensation c) heat regulation d) excretion e) secretion f) absorption
8. Dermatology is the study of the skin, its nature, structure, functions, diseases, and treatment.
9. A lesion of the skin is a structural change in the tissues caused by injury or disease.
10. Acne is a chronic inflammatory disorder of the sebaceous glands.
11. a virus infection commonly called fever blisters
12. congenital absence of melanin pigment of the body, including the skin, hair, and eyes
13. A mole is a small, brownish spot, or blemish, on the skin.

Chapter 22
REMOVING UNWANTED HAIR
(Answers to Questions on Page 500)

1. Hirsuties means hairiness, or superfluous hair. It is recognized by the growth of hair in unusual amounts or locations, as on the faces of women.
2. a) permanent b) temporary
3. The first effective technique of permanent hair removal invented was electrolysis. This technique was devised by the ophthalmologist Charles E. Michel.
4. Thermolysis is the method of hair removal using high-frequency or alternating current, developed in 1924.
5. the blend method
6. a) shaving b) tweezing c) depilatories
7. a) lower eyelids b) inside the ears c) nostrils
8. The shortwave method, also known as the thermolysis method, is the quickest method of permanent hair removal.
9. a) Test the temperature of the heated wax. b) Use caution so the wax does not contact the eyes. c) Do not use a wax depilatory under the arms, over warts, on moles, abrasions, irritated or inflamed skin.

Chapter 23
CELLS, ANATOMY, AND PHYSIOLOGY
(Answers to Questions on Page 528)

1. As the basic functional units, the cells carry on all life processes. Cells also have the ability to reproduce, providing new ones for growth and replacement of worn and injured tissues.
2. As long as cells receive an adequate supply of food, oxygen, and water; eliminate waste products; and are favored with proper temperature, they will grow and thrive.
3. Metabolism is a complex chemical process whereby the body cells are nourished and supplied with the energy needed to carry on their many activities.
4. The brain controls the body; the heart circulates the blood; the lungs supply oxygen to the blood; the liver removes toxic products of digestion; the kidneys excrete water and waste products; and the stomach and intestines aid in the digestion of food.
5. Systems are groups of organs that cooperate for a common purpose, namely the welfare of the entire body.
6. Anatomy is the study of the structure of the body and what it is made of, for example, bones, muscles, and skin.
7. Physiology is the study of the functions or activities performed by the structures of the body.
8. Histology is the study of the minute structural parts of the body, such as hair, nails, sweat glands, and oil glands.
9. to give shape and support to the body; to protect various internal structures and organs; to serve as attachments for muscles and act as levers to produce body movements; to produce various blood cells in the red bone marrow; to store various minerals, such as calcium, phosphorus, magnesium, and sodium
10. The muscular system covers, shapes, and supports the skeleton. Its function is to produce all movements of the body. The muscular system consists of over 500 muscles, large and small, comprising 40 to 50% of the weight of the human body.
11. a) to learn how to administer scalp and facial services for the client's benefit b) to know what effects these treatments have on the nerves in the skin and scalp and on the body as a whole
12. It keeps the blood moving within the circulatory system.
13. The blood is composed of red and white corpuscles, blood platelets, and plasma.
14. Lymph is a colorless, watery fluid that is derived from the plasma of the blood, mainly by filtration through the capillary walls into the tissue spaces.
15. a) exocrine, or duct glands b) endocrine, or ductless glands

16. a) kidneys b) liver c) skin d) large intestine e) lungs
17. With each respiratory, or breathing, cycle an exchange of gases takes place. During inhalation, oxygen is absorbed into the blood; carbon dioxide is expelled during exhalation.
18. The digestive system changes food into soluble form, suitable for use by the cells of the body.

Chapter 24
ELECTRICITY AND LIGHT THERAPY
(Answers to Questions on Page 544)

1. Electricity is a form of energy that produces magnetic, chemical, and heat effects.
2. A conductor is a substance that permits electric current to pass through it easily.
3. A nonconductor or insulator is a substance that resists the passage of an electric current, such as rubber, silk, dry wood, glass, cement, or asbestos.
4. Direct current (DC) is a constant, even-flowing current, traveling in one direction. It produces a chemical reaction.
5. Alternating current (AC) is a rapid and interrupted current, flowing first in one direction and then in the opposite direction. It produces a mechanical action.
6. It is a constant and direct current, reduced to a safe, low-voltage level. Chemical changes are produced when this current is used.
7. The positive pole produces acidic reactions. The negative pole produces alkaline reactions.
8. The positive pole: a) closes the pores b) soothes the nerves c) decreases blood supply.
9. The negative pole: a) opens the pores b) stimulates the nerves c) increases blood supply.
10. if it causes pain or discomfort; if the face is very florid; and if the client has many gold-filled teeth, high blood pressure, broken capillaries, or pustular conditions of the skin

Chapter 25
CHEMISTRY
(Answers to Questions on Page 580)

1. A basic knowledge of modern chemistry is an essential requirement for an intelligent understanding of the multitude of products and cosmetics currently used in the salon.
2. Organic chemistry is the branch of chemistry that deals with all substances in which carbon is present. Inorganic chemistry is the branch of chemistry that deals with all substances that do not contain carbon.
3. a) solids b) liquids c) gases
4. A physical change refers to a change in the form of a substance, without the formation of any new substance. For example, ice, a solid substance, melts at a certain temperature and becomes a liquid.
5. A chemical change is one in which a new substance or substances are formed, having properties different from the original substances. For example, when you mix hydrogen peroxide into a para dye, a chemical change occurs.
6. The pH of a substance is a chemical measure of its acidity or alkalinity.
7. a) anionic b) cationic c) nonionic d) ampholytic
8. They are the composition of numerous parallel fibers of hard keratin in the cortex.
9. a) salt bonds called S bonds b) hydrogen bonds called H bonds c) disulfide bonds called S-S bonds
10. Permanent waving lotion causes the cuticle of the hair to swell and the imbrications to open, allowing the solution to penetrate into the cortex. The solution breaks the disulfide bonds found within the cortex.
11. The base of an oxidation tint is composed of aromatic (fragrant) compounds obtained almost exclusively from coal. They are synthetic organic ingredients that when mixed with an oxidizer work with the couplers to create artificial pigment. The couplers are ingredients added to obtain certain colors, preserve and stabilize the product, and improve the resulting condition of the hair shaft. When you mix oxidation tints with the oxidizing agent (hydrogen peroxide), an alkaline reaction creates a chemical process, which causes the cortex to swell.
12. a) powders b) solutions c) suspensions d) emulsions e) ointments f) soaps
13. It is no longer used as a skin sanitizer because of current classification as a hazardous chemical due to its ability to kill living tissue.
14. Depilatories contain detergents to strip the sebum from the hair and adhesives to hold the chemicals to the hair shaft for the 5 to 10 minutes necessary to remove the hair.
15. a) cleansing cream b) wrinkle treatments c) moisturizers d) massage cream
16. Astringents are designed to remove oil accumulation on the skin.
17. Many foundations contain barrier agents, such as UV inhibitors, cellulose derivatives, and silicone.

Chapter 26
THE SALON BUSINESS
(Answers to Questions un Page 599)

1. When planning to open a salon, give careful consideration to every aspect of running a business, including location, written agreements, business regulations, laws, insurance, salon operation, record keeping, and salon policies.

2. A salon can be owned and operated by an individual, a partnership, or a corporation.

3. They are used to determine income, expenses, profit, or loss; to assess the value of the salon for prospective buyers; to arrange a bank loan or financing; for reports on income tax, Social Security, unemployment and disability insurance, accidents, and for percentage payments of gross income required in some leases.

4. a) consumption supplies b) retail supplies

5. Since the reception area is the first thing clients see, it should be attractive, appealing, and comfortable.

6. Good telephone habits and techniques make it possible for the salon owner and cosmetologist to increase business and improve relationships with clients and suppliers.

7. a) Be familiar with the merits and benefits of each service and product. b) Adapt your approach and technique to meet the needs of each client. c) Be self-confident. d) Generate interest and desire, which are the steps leading to a sale. e) Never misrepresent your service or product. f) Use tact when selling to a client. g) Don't underestimate the client or the client's intelligence. h) To sell a product or service, deliver a sales talk in a relaxed, friendly manner and, if possible, demonstrate its use. i) Recognize the right psychological moment to close any sale. Once the client has offered to buy, quit selling—don't oversell, except to praise the client for the purchase and assure her that she will be happy with it.

8. all activities that promote a favorable impression on the public

9. a pleased client

NOTES

NOTES

NOTES

NOTES

NOTES

NOTES

NOTES

NOTES

NOTES

NOTES

NOTES

NOTES

NOTES

NOTES

NOTES

NOTES

NOTES

NOTES

NOTES